D0722031

REJUVENATION: *The History of an Idea*

REJUVENATION

The History of an Idea

ERIC J. TRIMMER, M.B., B.S.

SOUTH BRUNSWICK
NEW YORK: A. S. BARNES AND COMPANY

REJUVENATION. © Eric J. Trimmer 1967. First American edition published 1970 by A. S. Barnes and Company, Inc., Cranbury, New Jersey 08512.

Library of Congress Catalogue Card Number: 70-83391

SBN 498 07502 8

Printed in the United States of America

Contents

Illustrations

ACKNOWLEDGEMENTS

The illustrations are reproduced by courtesy of the following: the Wellcome Historical Medical Museum, 1, 2, 5, 13,
14, 15; the Wellcome Trustees, 3, 4, 6, 7, 8, 9; the Royal
Society of Medicine Photographic Department, 10, 11; the
Editor, *Family Doctor*, 16.

1

A Matter for Experiment

Man is essentially an experimental animal and a fair indication of his degree of sophistication is the extent to which he will experiment in an attempt to control his environment and the forces it seems are constantly working on him for good and evil.

A natural enough characteristic of mankind too is to look upon the process of living as something essentially good and natural while the process of dying is assumed to be something essentially bad and unnatural. Or at least an event to mourn and if possible to postpone. There are simple enough reasons behind such basic convictions. In primitive society the active male represented power, measured usually in terms of protection and production, while the reproductive female held in her grasp the solution to the tribe's existence by the replacement of those seen to be ageing, non-productive and dying.

In many small communities the death of an individual would appear as a great calamity and therefore a very bad thing. If many died at the same time, as in epidemics, the whole community might disintegrate. And so experimental man thought about death a great deal and tried to avoid its "badness" in various ways. An obvious answer was to experiment with ways of prolonging his active life, and that of his womenfolk. Thus the first ideas in the history of rejuvenation were evolved. To some extent the methods which sophisticated mankind has used to solve basic problems have been quite similar to those used by the earliest societies. Death and the cheating of death is often looked upon as a trick by the savage. In rejuvenation today, magic, or trickster beliefs are popular. An example of this mystical and magical rejuvenation is seen, for example, in the quest for magic elixirs and even fountains of youth.

Perhaps a rather more sophisticated approach is to look at old age, senility, non-productivity and death as the result of malevolent demons craving to claim mankind. Or accepting such calamities as a punishment for sins committed. A simple extension of this idea, when moral sins are less worrying to a society, is to lay the unpleasantness of later years, that rejuvenation will presumably help us to escape, at the door of more tangible evils. For instance, senility may be thought to be due to nutritional mistakes or dietary indiscretions. This rationale too has its modern counterpart.

A fairly high degree of experimental control of the basic business of preventing ageing, or restoring youth, is the use of substances that for the want of a better word we call drugs. The word drug, of course, has no precise meaning. It can be anything from aspirin to arrowroot, or from the juice of the autumn crocus to cortisone. Drugs evolved naturally by simple extensions from pure magic and although a tremendous amount of magic still clings to drugs, mankind eventually came to realize, by experiment, that they sometimes also had strictly predictable and repeatable therapeutic effects, quite divorced from the Art of Magic.

Some of the oldest rejuvenation literature is concerned with drugs. The Edwin Smith papyrus tells us of a simple drug method of transforming an old man into a youth of twenty. It consisted of hemoyet fruit and khar dried in the sun and later boiled up with water to make either an ointment or a *cataplasma*. This was spread on the body, and was "found effective in myriads of cases". It not only removed all blemishes and disfigurements from the skin but also cured "all signs of age, and all weakness that flesh was heir to". It does not seem so very far removed from the modern beautician's face pack.

More common perhaps, in all rejuvenating techniques popular

in ancient times, is the employment of complicated ritual in which magic and medicine are intricately interwoven. The classical example of this in antiquity comes to us in the story of the rejuvenation of Aeson. It will be remembered that when the *Argo* returned from her triumphal voyage she bore an unexpected prize. Jason had not only obtained the Golden Fleece but also a bride, Medea, who had helped him so much on his voyage of adventure. But, of course, the Argonauts had been away from Iolkos for a long time and Jason found his father Aeson senile and unable to leave his home or take part in any of the festivities planned to celebrate the glorious return.

Jason was, we are told, profoundly affected by his father's condition. In his agony he appealed to Medea to use her magical powers to take some of the years of his own life and add them to that of his father's. Understandably perhaps the young bride would hear none of this, and rebuked her spouse: "Your words are impious, even Hekate herself cannot do this". As an afterthought, however, she agreed to try and rejuvenate the old man with the aid of the Three-faced Goddess and her Grant.

Medea first of all invoked the aid of Mother Earth, Hekate and Black Night to help her to "find juices, by whose aid the old man will be renewed" and returned to the vigour of his earlier years. Conjuring up her winged dragons she drove over Tempe, Ossa, Pelion, Othrys, Pindus, Olympus, Apidanus, Enipeus, Spercleius, Peneus and Boebe, in search of roots and grasses with rejuvenating properties. Although it took her nine whole days, ultimately she was successful. So powerful were the herbs she had gathered that their very smell affected Medea's dragons, who sloughed off their old skins and became young again.

When Medea finally returned with her drugs, however, these alone were not relied upon to bring about the much-desired rejuvenation. First she built two altars of turf, one to Hekate and the other to Youth. In the nearby ditches a complicated religio-magical ceremony was performed. First the turfs were soaked with the blood of a black ram, then with wine and then with milk. After suitable prayers the aged Aeson was brought out and laid down on to a bed of herbs. Because the ceremony was secret Jason and his attendants were only allowed to watch at a distance as the altars were illuminated with flaming brands and Medea purified the old man with fire, water and sulphur.

While this ceremony was going on a selection of the herbs Medea had procured were being boiled together with "pebbles from the farthest Orient, hoarfrost gathered under the moon, wings and flesh of the *infamous* horned owl, entrails of a werewolf, the skin of the Cynyphian water snake, liver of a long lived stag, the head of a crow nine centuries old and a thousand other things". Medea stirred her brew with an old dried up olive branch and watched, presumably with some satisfaction, as it began to sprout leaves, flowers and even bore fruit. As the cauldron bubbled over, the earth on to which the liquid fell, grew green and bore flowers.

Judging that the *moment critique* had arrived Medea cut Aeson's throat and allowed him to bleed profusely. Then she made the old man drink the potent broth and infused it also into his wound. The effects were immediate. His beard and hair changed from grey to black. He lost his lean and withered look and his limbs filled out into youthful lines. All in all Aeson returned to a physical state enjoyed forty years previously.[1]

The various stages in this classic rejuvenation and the materia medica involved in Ovid's story are highly relevant to the whole history of ideas in rejuvenation. Jason only wanted his father brought back to youth so that he could be rescued from the infirmity of age. Sexual rejuvenation was not requested of Medea, and so Satyricon was absent from the recipe. There seems no doubt that Medea was an extremely strong and resourceful person. These personality traits are present in contemporary practitioners of the Art.

The very latest ideas on rejuvenation have had to await the development of a high degree of experimentation by man— graced with the sub-titles biochemistry, pathology, pharmacology and endocrinology. In all likelihood there is much more that experimental man will find to do, with advantage, in the years to come. And many more forceful characters will certainly emerge to carry out the treatment.

2

Plant Remedies

The development of the idea that rejuvenation and other medical procedures could be accomplished with the aid of plants is probably evidence of a fair degree of sophistication in the evolution of primitive societies. The earliest common folklore belief is, as Garrison points out,[2] essentially animistic. Broadly this supposes the world to be inhabited with many invisible forces that are responsible for all disease and death. Gradually primitive man elaborated methods, quite logical in his own conception of things, that might be expected to influence these forces.

The conviction that a spirit life exists *pari passu* with materialistic existence was probably commonplace in prehistoric man, as it is with contemporary tribal societies. Perhaps the experience of a dreaming world alongside waking existence stimulated this hypothesis. The spirit world, once accepted as an experience shared by all, soon became peopled in men's imagination with spirits of good and evil. In the beginning they were probably very much like themselves, and it was instinctive to try to cajole or placate them with sacrifices or offerings.

Once this conception of the individual's medical fate crystallized, man started to worry about other men being perhaps more influential with the spirits who were responsible for health or disease. Increased imaginative experience probably gave gradual rise to the idea in primitive society that the spirits of the dead influenced the lives of the living and that these spirits might emanate from living and non-living sources.

Once this presumptive stage was reached in the evolution of what is best thought of as Folk Medicine, the whole comprehension of the cause of disease became sufficiently complicated to warrant the natural development in the community of an expert qualified to deal with it: whether this took the form of a witch doctor, a wisewoman, or a herb doctor was immaterial. Someone appears on the scene, skilled in medical lore and available to the community.

Those chosen for this important task, as well as being temperamentally suited to handling the spiritual or psychological role effectively, also had to be versed in food and herb lore. They knew what was safe for cattle and men to eat, and also what was toxic or poisonous. The extent to which these branches of primitive medicine are intertwined is demonstrated by the survival of the Greek word *pharmacos* in our language, for it describes those who enjoy a knowledge of drugs and their actions. The ancient Greek Spring Festival of the Thargelia demonstrates a primitive fear of the sorcerer. Every year two outcasts of the community were reserved as scapegoats and designated Pharm Kos, to be publicly and ceremonially beaten, stoned to death or drowned.[3]

A recent study of folk medicine[4] and doctoring in rural Greece points out that in that area both the doctor and the folk-medicine practitioner are still held in rather low esteem and regarded with suspicion. But elsewhere in the world the practice of all medical arts gradually gathered momentum.

In early days, as far as the history of rejuvenation is concerned, a fairly heavy undertow or magic swept many practitioners out of their depth. And perhaps the deepest and most persistently fallacious magic adhered for years to the plant mandrake (*Mandragora officinarum*) of the potato order, (*Solancea*), and native of Spain, Sicily, Crete, Syria and North Africa. It is an inoffensive weed with a short stem, oval leaves and when the flowers appear they are in the form of a solitary purple corolla. The fruit is a fleshy orange-coloured berry. The root of the mandrake is often forked and fleshy like that of an imperfectly grown carrot, and if the whole plant is viewed with eyes fairly heavily clouded with conviction, its general configuration might be said to resemble that of a man or a woman.

In very early times mandrake was used as an emetic, or in smaller doses as a narcotic drug, and in the first century it was recommended that wine made from mandrake should be given to those about to be "cut" or cauterized, and Guthrie suggests this as the first reference to the use of surgical anaesthesia.[5] Shakespeare was cognisant of this action, for Cleopatra cries for a draught of mandragora to make her sleep while Anthony is away and the "drowsy syrup" of mandrago is mentioned in *Othello* coupled, therapeutically, with the syrup of poppy or opium.

As might be expected, smaller doses than those necessary to produce sleep or anaesthesia are capable of inducing a state of mild intoxication or confusion. It may be that this effect is responsible for the plant's place in the history of rejuvenation. In many cases rejuvenation in the sexual sphere is more apparent than real. Quite often what appears to be rejuvenation is really a temporary release from oppressive restrictions or social *mores*. Havelock Ellis pointed this out in his early writings on sex[6] with reference to alcohol, although he tended to opine that a direct aphrodisiac effect was experienced by women with this drug, and this is also suggested by Chaucer.

> A likerous mouth moste have a likerous tayle—
> This knowen lechours by experience.
> (Prologue to the *Wife of Bath's Tale*)

The classical example of mandrake as a rejuvenator, however, comes from biblical writings of the Old Testament. It is interesting to speculate on the psychological make-up of Jacob, Rachel and Leah. It will be remembered that these sisters were daughters of Laban, Jacob's uncle. Leah was "tender eyed" but Rachel "beautiful and well favoured", and it was with the latter that her cousin fell in love. Laban was, the Bible tells us, something of a rogue. Jacob was living in his house and, determined to marry Rachel, he agreed to serve Laban for seven years for his daughter's hand. The bargain was struck and the deed eventually redeemed.

Laban, however, is said to have tricked Jacob into sleeping with Leah on his marriage night and excused his ruse by saying that in his country the youngest child must not be married first; nevertheless he promised Rachel also, after a week's marriage to Leah.

Simultaneously married to the two sisters, trouble was inevitable. Leah bore Jacob four sons, but Rachel was barren and so she decided to put a practice, not uncommon at the time, into effect. This was to encourage her husband to cohabit with her maid Bilhah, and bring up any children of the union as her own. Naturally enough, this directed Jacob's attention from sister Leah until she countered by giving her maid Zilpah to her husband in the same way.

Both servant-girls bore Jacob more sons, and the rejuvenating principle of mandrake comes into history in the following way. One of Leah's sons was helping with the harvest, and while in the field he came across some mandrakes growing. Presumably, even at this time, the valuable properties of the plant were widely known, for the boy brought them home excitedly to his mother. Rachel begged Leah to give her some, and one gathers that she did so. Leah greeted Jacob with the words, "Thou must come in unto me for surely I have hired thee with thy son's mandrakes". Whether or not she partook of the root herself, or gave it to Jacob is not made clear in *Genesis*, but apparently the rejuvenation worked, for Leah conceived another son and subsequently further children. Later, of course, perhaps with the aid of Leah's mandrakes, Rachel managed to conceive as well.

Mandrake is still said to be used for its narcotic and rejuvenating properties in Africa and the East. But in the West many curious tales grew up about the mandrake. One was that extreme care must be taken relative to harvesting the root, as the plant was said to emit a terrible shriek, liable to drive men mad, or worse still, kill those who dug it up. Early writers suggested getting the plant out of the ground by the expedient of tying it to a dog's tail, plugging one's ears and then kicking the unfortunate animal, who therefore unwittingly harvested it. Thus the dangerous shrieks were avoided. An old English belief that mandrakes grow particu-

larly well under gallows "nourished by the exhalations from executed criminals" would seem to make its culture extremely
difficult, and in fact may have given the plant its popular name of
"Rarity".

That mandrake was a rare plant led to various imitations being
made, usually from wild bryony. This was well known by Dioscorides, the Greek army surgeon who served under Nero (A.D.
54-68), and who, taking advantage of his facilities for travel,
made a study of plants and their properties. Thus he became the
first medical botanist and his knowledge was used with little
alteration for sixteen centuries. Although Dioscorides recommended mandrake wine for insomnia or pain, he was against many of
the "ridiculous" and "doltish tales" about the plant as far as the
effects of its supposed lethal or manic properties with regard to its
harvesting.

One medical historian's opinion that mandrakes were therapeutically inert due to the fact that Andre Paré, the humanistic
surgeon of the sixteenth century, rejected them as a pre-operative
drug is not entirely valid.[7] The mandrake grown in Southern
Europe and the Levant may well be a very different plant from
the pharmacological point of view from the one grown in colder
climates. It is well known that, as far as alkaloid content, plants
vary profoundly between varieties in the same species. Details of
cultivation, daily hours of sunlight in which they grow, and many
other factors are also capable of making gross variations in the yield
of active principle, even in the same species of plant. Treatment
after harvesting, storage and method of preparation for use vary
the therapeutic effect of vegetable substances as well.

One prominent botanist [8] draws attention to the fact that mandrake roots are very similar to those of belladonna, and that they
contain an alkaloid called mandragorine. In all probability, she
feels, this is identical with atropine or hyoscyamine. If this is the
case some of the supposedly "ridiculous" effects of mandrake root
may well be true. It is well known that large doses of atropine
have profound effects on psychic function. High doses produce
symptoms suggestive of alcoholic inebriation which pass, with
increasing dosage, into deep sedation. While in the mildly

intoxicated condition with atropine, a sense of exaltation is pronounced, and this effect tends to be very prolonged.

One way in which quacks produced "mandrakes" to sell to their customers was to

> carve upon plants, while still green, male and female forms, inserting millet or barley seeds in such parts as they desire the likeness of human hair to grow on: then, digging a hole in the ground, they place the plants therein, covering them with sand, till such time as the little seeds have stricken root, which it is said, would be perfectly effected within twenty days at farthest. After this, disinterring the plants, these impostors with a sharp cutting knife, so dexterously carve, pare and slip [sic] the little filaments of the seeds as to make them resemble the hair which grows upon the various parts of the human body.[9]

Moving from mandrakes to other plants held to be rejuvenating from times of antiquity onwards, the most ancient are the orchids. It is difficult to argue why this enormous family of plants suggested themselves as therapeutic aids to early practitioners of folk medicine or doctors. As far as the terrestrial orchids are concerned, the doctrine of signatures may be evoked. Because the orchids intertwine themselves with great tenacity to strong trees, often as we shall see later themselves venerated with reference to rejuvenation, the reasoning is that orchids too have great power and strength on this score. As far as sexual rejuvenation is concerned the very act of intertwining suggests sexual congress, but it is hard to apply this theory to the tuberous roots of the terrestrial orchids. The best that can be argued would be a similarity between the shape of these tubercules and the shape of the testes. Orchid, of course, is the Latin for testicle, and this argument might be extended to cover the pseudo-bulbs of terrestrial orchids which have a very similar shape.

It would seem highly likely that such theories are more fancy than fact and in all probability the wide distribution of orchids throughout the world (the *Orchidacae* is the largest family of the monocotyledons, including the grasses), and the apparently tempting nature of their plump tuberosities encouraged men to use them as an experimental foodstuff or medicine. Physiological effects were presumably noticed and another rejuvenant was born.

The early purple orchid (*Orchis mascula*), has many local names that suggest a connection with sexual rejuvenation, and in Europe from the Middle Ages onwards herbals contained instructions for making water of satyrion. Hieronymous Braunschweig's *Liber de ante distillandi*, translated into English by Laurence Andrew, told how this water if taken in one and a half ounce doses night and morning, "causeth great heat, therefore it giveth lust unto the workes of generacyon and multiplycaton of sperms". In the seventeenth century the orchid was made into an infusion with wine in New England and John Josselyn in 1672 saw "a wanton woman . . . compounding an Amorous Cup" with orchid root, "which wrought the desired effect". Back in England it was boldly stated that "enough orchids grew in Cobham Park in Kent to pleasure all the seamen's wives in Rochester".[10] For all this it was not the natural product but the dried powdered orchid root which really put orchids on the map as far as rejuvenation is concerned.

The properties of salep, (a powder made from the tuberosities), gradually established a world-wide reputation as a restorative and rejuvenant. At first it was extensively used in the East, generally imported from the Levant, but in 1760 the French chemist, Geoffroy, discovered the powder's composition and showed how it could be made from French orchids. The Germans quickly followed suit and soon the English were making their own salep from common terrestrial orchids.

A Mr. Mault of Rochdale explained the technique:

Wash the fresh roots in water and separate the outer brown skin or dip them in hot water and rub the skin off with a cloth. Spread the blanched roots on a tin plate and bake them in the oven from six to ten minutes during which time they will lose their milky richness and acquire the transparency of bones. Remove them from the oven and leave them in the air for several days to harden, or they can be left to harden for a few hours in the oven. Powder as required.[11]

Salep was, however, hard to powder and usually had to be ground between millstones. Almost every country in the Near and Middle East produced vast quantities of salep, and in the middle of the nineteenth century well over three hundred tons were exported from Smyrna alone.

Usually salep was taken dissolved in water or mixed with an alcoholic drink. The latter aided the solution of the powder and presumably made the mucilaginous solution more palatable. It was served as an alternative to coffee in many fashionable coffee houses in the eighteenth century and one "Salep House" existed in Fleet Street in London.

Whether salep was anything more than a craze or had a real rejuvenating property is rather difficult to decide. The belief is one of the greatest antiquity and is even recorded in mythological terms. Certain species of the *Orchidacae* are named *Satyrion*, which suggests they were responsible for the behaviour of the Satyrs. The extensive production of salep on a world-wide basis also seems significant, were it not for evidence of other substances enjoying, for a considerable time, a totally unwarranted favour.

From the point of view of science salep is rather a disappointment. Pharmacologically it is mainly a mucilaginous demulcent and as such is only very partially digested and for the most part excreted unchanged in the faeces. In the fresh state, however, orchid roots contain a volatile oil of uncertain composition together with an unidentified nitrogenous substance. Altogether there is too little pharmaceutical evidence to reject orchids having a rejuvenating or restorative property out of hand and perhaps further pharmacological study is indicated.

Another plant that has an underground foodstore and also developed a universal reputation as an aphrodisiac, and a rejuvenant is the root of the *Convolvulus batatas*, or sweet potato. It is possible that the doctrine of signatures may be here applied too. For this plant's natural twisting habit suggests a parasite clasping a tree with its tendrils. And this in folk lore is always perceived as a man embracing a woman.[12]

The origin of this plant remains obscure, and claims have been made for the Incas of Peru and the inhabitants of the West Indies as its first cultivators. Above the ground, it presents itself as a climbing perennial not unlike the common bindweed of the hedgerows. The sweet potato is intolerant of frosts but is widely cultivated in Japan, China, the South Sea Islands, Australia and New Zealand. It was imported quite early into these islands and Shakespearian mention of the potato refers to the *Convolvulus batatas*.

John Gerard, the barber surgeon, who was appointed "herbalist" to James I, cultivated over a thousand different varieties of herbs in his garden at Holborn, London, and described how he tried to grow the sweet potato in his garden at the "Exchange in London", but found they would not flower and rotted during the cold winter months. He also gives many other interesting sidelights on London in the sixteenth century, for example wild flowers growing in the ditches of Piccadilly and marigolds in the marshy ground round Paddington.

Sweet potatoes were abroad grown mainly as a food and at one time were a staple item in the dietary of the Maoris. As a rejuvenator, however, they had to be compounded into a sweetmeat or comfit.

Although sweet potatoes have always been a comparative rarity in Britain either as a food or rejuvenant, a common plant, sea holly or *Eryngium Maritimum*, surprisingly perhaps won for itself a reputation as an aphrodisiac and rejuvenant. The roots, in Elizabeth's England, were candied and in all probability were the "kissing comfits" of Falstaff. An apothecary from Colchester by the name of Robert Burton was said to have made them popular and Colchester Comfits used to be presented periodically to Royalty.[13]

Gerard thought that "condited" or sugar-preserved Eryngos were good for "old and aged people that are consumed with old age". His recipe for making them was as follows:

Refine sugar fit for the purpose and take a pound of it, the white of an egge, and a pinte of cleer water, boile them together and scum it, then let it boile until it be come to good strong syrrup, and when it is boiled, as it cooleth adde thereto a saucer full of rose water, a spoone full of Cinnamon water, and a grain of muske, which have been infused together the night before, and now strained: into which syrrup being more than halfe cold, put in your roots to soke and infuse untill the next day: your roots being ordered in manner hereafter following:

These your roots being washed and picked, must be boiled in faire
water by the space of foure houres, til'they be soft: then must they be
pilled clean as ye pil parsneps, & the pith must be drawn out at the
end of the root.: but if there be any whose pith cannot be drawn out
at the end, then you must slit them and so take it out: these you must
also keep from much handling, that they may be clean: let them remain in the syrrup till the next day, and then set them on the fire in
a faire broad pan untill they be very hot, but let them not boile at all:
let them remain over the fire an hour or more, remooving them
easily in the pan from one place to another with a wooden slice.
This done, have in a readiness great cap or royall papers, whereupon
strow some sugar, upon which lay your roots, having taken them
out of the pan. These papers you must put into a stouve or hot-house
to harden: but if you have not such a place, lay them before a good
fire: in this manner if you condite your roots there is not any that
can prescribe you a better way. And thus you may condite any other
root whatsoever, which will not only be exceeding delicate, but
very wholesome, and effectual against the diseases above named.

Comfits were also recommended as a sexual rejuvenant by the
author of the *Perfumed Garden:* "If therefore a man will passionately give himself up to the enjoyment of coition without undergoing too great fatigue he must live on strengthening food,
exciting comfits. . . ."[14]

Eryngo plants, as might be expected, grow along the seashore,
to a height of one and a half feet, bearing blue flowers. The botanical title is derived from a Greek word meaning to belch, and both
the flowers and the roots were well thought of for many centuries
as diuretics and diaphoretics as well as for their stimulating properties. In Sweden at one time the flower shoots were eaten like
asparagus. Sea holly was widely used throughout Europe and
was especially regarded in Arabia. According to Loudon, "English
grooms often mix the dried plant with the corn they give to
stallions in the covering season".

The active principle in Eryngo has not been identified. Apparently the root has a definite pharmacological effect, for its actions
are diaphoretic, diuretic and expectorant. Eryngo sweetmeats
were once very popular in the treatment of tuberculosis. As far
as the diuretic effect is concerned it is possible that this is due to
the presence of a volatile oil that irritates the kidney. It is well

known that several naturally occurring volatile oils in large doses produce pelvic congestion and this may possibly be why sea holly gained a reputation as a sexual rejuvenant.

Another plant well thought of as a rejuvenant is Rocket or *Hesperis matronalis*. Rocket is a member of the large family *Cruciferae* and many of this non-poisonous order of plants are eaten in the form of salads. The suggestion that the antiscorbutic factor of Rocket might be the reason for its popularity in rejuvenation— and certainly anyone suffering from severe Vitamin C deficiency would benefit from it—falls because almost all salad vegetables also contain this essential vitamin.

Once again there is every likelihood that Rocket contains an unidentified substance with a strong pharmacological action. A large meal of Rocket-leaves causes vomiting. While the active principle involved remains unknown it is quite impossible to be dogmatic as to whether or not the plant is of real value as a rejuvenant. The fact remains that these properties of Rocket were well thought of by the Romans, and persist to this day, and are recommended in an amusing book on Rejuvenating Recipes.[15] Norman Douglas, its main author, who lived to be well over eighty, will probably be remembered as the founder of the Capri school of writers and author of the controversial novel *Southwind*. He died, Graham Greene tells us, "after a life consistently open, tolerant, unashamed! 'Ill spent' it has been called by the kind of judges whose condemnation is the highest form of praise. In a sense he had created Capri: there have been suicides, embezzlements, rapes, thefts, funerals and processions which would not have happened exactly that way if Douglas had not existed".

Greene thought it was fitting that Norman Douglas should spend his last days compiling a collection of rejuvenating recipes for "he had enjoyed varied forms of love, left a dozen or so living tokens of it here and there. . . . One remembers the old gypsy family from Northern Italy who had travelled all the way to Capri to spend an afternoon with Douglas and exhibit to him another grandchild". This is surely an extraordinary and possibly unique form of praise for a man who began his literary career as a third secretary at Her Majesty's Embassy in Saint Petersburg, writing a report on the Pumice Stone Industry of the Lipari Islands. The dish that appears in *Venus in the Kitchen* contains twenty leaves of rocket, half a lettuce, and a clove of chopped garlic, served with French salad dressing.

It is interesting to note that there is another Rocket of a different type, the Sea Rocket or *Eruca Monitima*. This may be the "wild rocket" Nicholas Culpepper enthuses over in his classic seventeenth-century herbal, *The Physician's Guide to Plants* that "increases sperm" and also cures the bites of serpents, takes away "ill scent from the armpits" as well as "foul scars, blue spots and the markes of the small pox".

Nicholas Culpepper was apparently an extraordinary man, and was said to have "a bonnet as full of bees as a border of catmint on a bright, sunny morning".[16] He believed passionately in astrological botany, in other words the influence of the Heavens on the plant world, and, although only an apothecary, gave himself a gratuitous M.D. and set up in practice at Red Lion House, Spitalfields. This brought him into conflict with the College of Physicians to whom he referred as "a company of proud, insulting, domineering Doctors, whose wits were born above five hundred years before themselves".

But we must not judge his opinion of wild Rocket too harshly on the grounds of his eccentricity and apparent credulity, because here and there in the history of rejuvenation we come across small gobbets of scientific information that seem to make the reappraisal of plant-induced rejuvenation entirely necessary. A good example is found in the herb Fenugreek.

This has as its normal habitat the Eastern shores of the Mediterranean but is also widely cultivated in India, Africa, Egypt and Morocco. It also can be grown in these islands. The name is derived from *Foenum Graecum*, meaning Greek hay, and the plant was used for many years as an additive to hay and has been held in high repute by medical and paramedical practitioners as a rejuvenant, aphrodisiac and restorative since ancient Egyptian and Greco-Roman times.

In all probability the ancients first noticed the improvement to cattle when the two-foot-high annual herb, with its brilliant cherry red flowers was added to fodder, and eventually the plant and its seeds were included in the physician's therapeutic armamentarium. It would be tempting to shrug off the supposed properties of Fenugreek as just another fantasy of Green Medicine, were it not for the fact that it contains a rich oil closely resembling cod liver oil in composition. This would probably account for increased wellbeing in animals or man, who were short of vitamins A and D in their diet.

As far as rejuvenation proper is concerned, another substance found in Fenugreek is trimethylamine. This acts as a sex hormone in frogs, causing them to moult and prepare for mating. Dilute solutions of this substance increase flower production in certain plants and also have an effect on the development of certain plant tumours. As yet effects on man are not documented.

Before leaving even a superficial account of rejuvenation brought about with the aid of plant life, mention must be made of the part that trees play in this arena. It is interesting to note that there is little evidence of this in the "Great European families of Aryan stock" that Frazer refers to in the *Golden Bough*. These people, of course, worshipped trees before the advent of Christianity, and there are relics of tree-worship in many folk practices to this day. In all probability the custom pertaining to the May tree, and the maypole in Britain, the Whitsuntide birch tree in Russia, the Firtree Ceremonies of Midsummer in Sweden, and various tree spirit rites throughout the whole of Europe are atavistic evidence of ancient tree worship.

The more direct descendants of the ancient people of India, Africa, Arabia and certain South American countries elaborated quite a different attitude towards trees, and many species came to be looked upon as sources of rejuvenation and strength. The Durian tree, a handsome forest plant that grows to the height of seventy or eighty feet is an interesting example of this belief. Growing in such widespread areas as Sumatra, Java, the Philippines, the Malayan Peninsula and the Bay of Bengal, the tree produces a fruit the size of a large coconut with a hard, external husk. Inside are five oval seeds the size of chestnuts. They contain a cream-coloured gelatinous substance described by the explorer of the Malay Archipelago, Wallace, as being like "rich butter custard, highly flavoured with almonds . . . intermingled with wafts of flavour that calls to the mind cream cheese, onion sauce, brown sherry, and other incongruities . . . it is neither acid nor sweet, non juicy, yet one feels the want of a name for these qualities, for it is perfect as it is". Pharmacologically it remains a mystery, but it is much revered by the people who eat it to rejuvenate themselves.

The dried fruit of the Saw Palmetto which grows profusely along the south-eastern seaboard of the United States is likewise well thought of as a rejuvenative tonic to the tissues, especially those of the organs of reproduction. In this case although considerable knowledge of its constituents exists and a medicine is made from its seeds and used in respiratory disease, digestive disturbances, and as a nutritive tonic and aphrodisiac, the essential oils and alkaloids that may be involved in producing its therapeutic effects remain unidentified.

Of course there are many other examples of tree products having rejuvenating properties. Musk seeds are venerated in Egypt and India, the resin of the Mastic tree is still widely used in the East, the juice from the trunk of the date palm in Africa and Arabia. Exactly why certain products of individual trees have won this reputation, while many other indigenous to the various areas have not, is an unsolved mystery, unless those who partake of them as restoratives or for rejuvenation find that they work.

A story is told[17] of Gilgamish the hero of the Assyrians who sets out to find the herb "Old Man Becomes Young". Having been told that the plant grows at the bottom of the sea Gilgamish rows out in a boat, weighs himself with stones, sinks down into the Persian Gulf, picks it and then starts home, quest over, with the rejuvenating herb safe and sound. Unhappily, Assyria being as it is, Gilgamish fancied a swim on the way home and while he was cooling his tired body in a lake a snake devoured the plant. Thus the legend has it that snakes became immortal and man lost for ever his chance of rejuvenation.

This story is interesting in many ways, not the least being that Alex Comfort, possibly the most experienced gerontologist of our time, believes that certain fishes and reptiles do in fact age so slowly to be virtually ageless, or die in all probability not from senile changes but simply due to "fair wear and tear".[18]

The Indians too have a legend about plant rejuvenation, this time citing the soma plant which the famous surgeon-physician Sushruta describes so carefully. The plant grew, we are told,[19] in all climates in India from the Himalayas to the Indus, from the Punjab to Kashmir. The plant which looked "as beautiful as the moon" had fifteen leaves, one of which grew every day in the "lighted fortnight" of the moon, until the full complement was made up, and then dropped daily while the moon waned until eventually the stem was bare. The bulb of the soma plant has to be pricked with a golden needle to obtain its active principal, and the milky fluid collected in a golden vessel.

The rites of drinking the soma exudate were extremely carefully prescribed. An auspicious hour and day was suggested by the physician. Then the patient had to purge himself and rest in a comfortable, shady chamber. After the soma plant had been blessed the juice was extracted as previously described, and swallowed in one draught. Then the patient was instructed not to sleep, but to remain meditating.

In case the impression is given that this is an entirely folksy treatment, with suggestion as the only therapeutic agent at work, it must be noted that powerful physiological effects also occurred. Quite often severe diarrhoea and sickness followed the ingestion of soma. The practice was to proscribe food and after a few days the patient lost a considerable amount of weight. By the seventh day only "bare animation" could be detected in the patient, "the vital spark being retained by the potency of the soma".

Treatment was, however, only just beginning. But the eighth day "the skin becomes cracked, the teeth, nails and hair begin to fall out", and the clinical picture would seem to be not dissimilar to that seen in patients being treated with modern cytotoxic drugs. Once this state of debility had been reached the patient was bathed in a decoction of soma, and by the seventeenth day "new teeth, well formed, symmetrical, strong, hard and clean as a diamond", would appear. From then on, simple foodstuffs were added to an enriched milk diet and eventually "glossy and coral coloured fingernails resembling the new rising sun in lustre" appeared as well as black, shining hair. The skin took the hue of "lotus blossom" and the musculature showed a new and vigorous development.

The whole rejuvenation took seven weeks, during which time the patient was not permitted to look in the mirror and learned to renounce all "passions and anger".

Soma rejuvenation sounds a pretty alarming affair, but the Indians apparently thought it well worth the trouble, for it allowed whoever partook of it to "witness ten thousand summers on earth in the full enjoyment of youth" . . . maintaining such vigour and strength that it was "in no way inferior to the combined strength of a thousand rutting elephants." Even allowing for the natural exuberance of Sushruta this would seem impressive. India's most ancient scripture, the Rig Veda, the book of a thousand hymns, is less fanciful and merely says that after drinking the soma we are

> Immortal grown:
> We've entered into light
> And all the Gods have known.

The date of the writings of Sushruta has never been satisfactorily pegged. Many of the medicinal herbs described therein are still used in the Indian materia medica today, but there is no trace of the soma plant anywhere among India's luxuriant flora. Ilza Veith [20] feels that soma, like many other ancient plant extracts which have found a place in modern therapeutics, for example, rauwolfia serpentina, ephedrine and quinine, may be rediscovered one day. Then the "divine potion of eternal youth and tranquillity" may indeed become known to mankind.

Summarizing the position that plants hold in the history of rejuvenation is not easy. Obviously in the past they have held great favour, and it has only been possible to touch upon a few of the major successes in this short survey. How much they helped those who used them it is impossible to say. Often sexual rejuvenation was all that was asked of them and in many cases this seems to have been achieved. But perhaps the most important fact that emerges in even the most superficial analysis of plant-induced rejuvenation is the poverty of our knowledge of many of the active principles obtained from plants. Often the essential oils are not even named, and those that are have not been examined scientifically. The same applies to many of the alkaloids found in plant life and this seems to be a state of affairs quite unexpected in our professed scientific world of the twentieth-century.

3

Animal Products and Rejuvenation

Apart from the activities in the nineteenth and twentieth centuries of such practitioners as Metchnikoff, Steinach and Niehans, (*see* chapters 5, 6 and 7), much less use has been made of zoological raw material in the history of rejuvenation than of plant derivatives. There are, of course, ancient precedents for this, and the art and science of pharmacy is strongly and irrevocably interwoven with the atavisms of Green Medicine.

As far as European Medicine is concerned the position in the latter half of the seventeenth century can be gleaned from an appraisal of contemporary pharmacopoeias. Nicholas Culpepper devotes less than three pages to "Parts of living Creatures and Excrements", together with those "belonging to the Sea" in a book of 305 pages.[21] Other similar books of the *Physicians' Library* genre give like representation to zoological derivatives in medicine at this time.

Very few of the animal products described by Culpepper claimed any rejuvenating property. The brain of the hare roasted was thought good for "trembling", and also helped children to "breed teeth easily". Cataract, skin growing over the sight, responded to the "head of a coalblack cat burnt to ashes in a new pot and some of the ashes blown into the Eye", and a "head of a young Kite, (some countries call them Gleads and others Puttocks)", treated in the same way, was recommended for gout.

Crabs' eyes, incidentally nothing to do with crabs, being the concretions found in the stomachs of crayfish, a then common occupant of our streams and rivers, cured "the stone", and sheep's or goats' bladder burnt to ashes helped "diabetes and continual pissing".

Those who see evidence of sympathetic magic in seventeenth-century pharmacy in the giving of "the lunges of a fox well dried and not burned", as a "lung strengthener", are hard put to explain the "yard (penis) of a stag", recommended for "fluxes the bitings of enormous beasts".

The perusal of animal cures three centuries old reminds us that our forefathers suffered from the self-same diseases that our frames are heir to now. As well as the organic diseases, so confidently dealt with, for example, "that small triangular bone in the skull of a man, called *os triquerum*, so absolutely cures Falling Sickness that it will never come again", there was also a prevalence of psychosomatic illness. Alcoholism was treated by putting a live eel into the dipsomaniac's favourite tipple and allowing it to die therein. The patient quaffed the fluid and "never endured that sort of liquor again". Whey was used to treat depressive illnesses. Goose grease was used gynaecologically for "stiffness of the womb", and those whose amorous propensities had produced "running of the reins" were advised to eat young pigeons.

Fleeting reference is made in the *London Dispensatory* to sexual rejuvenation—"the brains of sparrows being eaten provoke lust exceedingly", but when more general rejuvenation cures were desired a complex pharmacological formula of a decidedly botanic character was preferred. An example was Laetificans Powder. "Take the flowers of Clove, Bazil, or the seeds thereof, Saffron Zedoory, Wood of Aloes, Cloves, Citron, Galanga, Mace, Nutmets, Styrax Calamitis, of each two drams and a half: Ivory, Aniseeds, Time, Epithimum, of each one dram: Bone of stag's heart, pearls, camphire of each half a dram: leaves of gold and silver, of each half a scruple: make into powder according to art".[21] This powder mixed in half a dram dose to any cordial electury not only caused "a merry heart" and helped digestion but also "keeps back old age".

As far as general rejuvenation is concerned the principle of giving aromatic and sweet flavoured "nervous simples" of a vegetable or herbal nature was almost standard practice well into the eighteenth century. Dr. John Quincey, famous as a medical lexicographer of some standing at this time, recommended such concoctions together with nervous cordials, as they "enter or soak into the nerves . . . whereupon their vibrations are invigorated . . . they comfort the heart, strengthen the brain, . . . and as constitution becomes weak by Age . . . are more and more helpful".[22]

But when sexual rather than general rejuvenation was sought the animal world came into greater use, and here some of the recommendations are of great antiquity. The Greeks apparently thought well of mussels, crabs, snails and eggs as sexual stimulants.[23] It is interesting to note that the authors of *Venus in the Kitchen*,[24] perhaps the only people who have extensively and seriously considered the rejuvenating properties of various foodstuffs, mention several recipes using just these ingredients. One curious recipe was the enigmatic *Snails à la C.C.C. N.111*. This involves boiling snails in salt water, sautéing them in olive oil together with onion, garlic, parsley and mushrooms, (all well favoured folklore rejuvenants in their own right), and then adding broth and strong red wine. The authors enthuse that "an old friend ate this dish in Bolgidinga when he was there and declares that he found himself at least ten years younger".

In antiquity many fantastic as well as practical rejuvenation devices enjoyed a certain popularity. Perhaps the most extraordinary of these concerned hippomanes.

The earliest mention of hippomanes occurs in Virgil's epic poem of action, manners and character, the *Aeneid*. Virgil, it will be remembered, was born on a farm near the town of Mantua, and in all probability the great national poet was well versed in natural lore. Strangely he mentioned hippomanes in association with a poison that the ill-starred heroine of the *Aeneid* concocts prior to her suicide.

> Herbs are brought, by moonlight mow'd
> With brazen scythes, big swol'n with milky juice

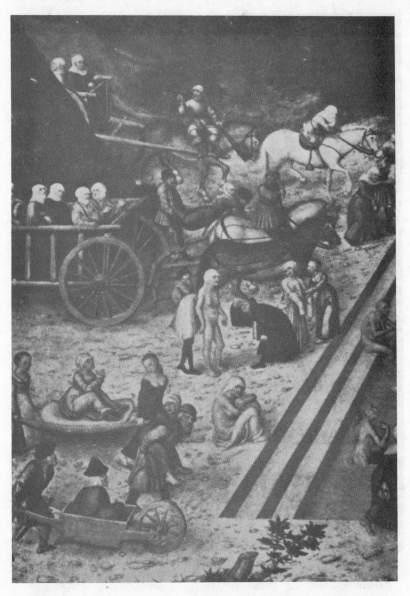

Detail from left-hand side of "The Fountain of Youth" by Lucas
Cranach the elder (1472–1553). The elderly are brought to the
edge of the fountain

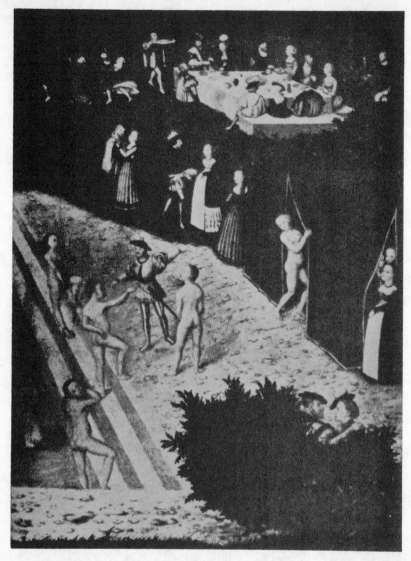

Detail from right-hand side of "The Fountain of Youth". After their rejuvenating bath patients are quick to enjoy their new found youth in many ways

Of curious poison and the fleshy knot
Torn from the forehead of a new foal'd colt [hippomanes],
To rob the mother's love.[24]

Rather later the satirical poet Juvenal mentions hippomanes in his sixth satire directed against the female sex that has been epitomized by the epithet "why marry, as long as there is rope to hang oneself with". A love potion containing hippomanes was prepared by Caesaria for administration to Cais:

Who, plucking from the forehead of a foal
The mother's love, infused it in the bowl:
The boiling blood ran hissing through his veins,
Till the mad vapour mounted to his brains.

Some two centuries later the famous Greek traveller and geographer Pausanias confirmed the rejuvenating property of hippomanes when he wrote about a statue of a horse in Olympia made by a magician, into the heads of which hippomanes had been worked. Although the craftsmanship of this statue was poor—it even had no tail—Pausanias tells us that

horses desire connection with this image not only in the spring but every day throughout the year, breaking their bridles or running away from their drivers, they rush into Altis and attack the horse in a manner much more furious than if it was the most beautiful mare. . . . Their hoofs indeed slip from the side of the image, but nevertheless they never cease neighing vehemently and leaping furiously on the figure till they are driven off by the whip or some other violent means, for till such methods are applied, it is impossible to disengage them from the brass.[25]

It would be easy to dismiss this extraordinary story as a piece of imaginative folklore, were it not for Pausanias's reputation as an accurate observer. Frazer appraises him as "a man made of common stuff", and his accuracy with regard to description is undisputed for "without him the ruins of Greece would for the most part be a labyrinth without a clue, a riddle without an answer".[25]

Strangely it seems that little interest has been shown in the scientific world with reference to hippomanes. Neither are folklore experts much involved with the belief (there is no mention of hippomanes in Dr. Wilfrid Bonser's admirable *Bibliography of Folklore*), although the word was used colloquially in English, the *Shorter Oxford English Dictionary* tells us, from the year 1601, and they held a considerable reputation as an aphrodisiac. Gradually a duplicated meaning became established and hippomanes also became known as "a mucous humour that runs from mares ahorsing".

Here and there in the history of medicine one comes across a fairly definite opinion that an animal product has a sound rejuvenating property. When this is voiced by someone essentially sensible and not prone to imaginative digressions it would seem worth remembering. Such a person was the eminent naturalist of the thirteenth century, Albertus Magnus, (Albert von Bollstädt). He was a Dominican monk who taught at Paris and Cologne and later became Bishop of Ratisbon. The making of strictly observational deductions was characteristic of his style and in his Tenth Book he declares, "all that is set down here is the result of our own experience, or has been borrowed from authors whom we know to have written what their personal experience has confirmed: for in these matters experience alone can give certainty".[26]

As a rejuvenant Albertus favoured the brains of partridge calcined into a powder and swallowed in red wine. This is of interest because partridge flesh has enjoyed a reputation as a restorative for many centuries. Platina, the historian of the political Popes of the fifteenth century, recommends the "flesh of the partridge which is of good and easy digestion" because it not only "strengthens the brain and facilitates conception" but also "arouses half-extinct desire for venereal pleasures".

Such writings stress again and again an inevitable mingling of sexual and general rejuvenation that seems to have occurred from the earliest times. The Chinese writer, Chin P'ing Mei, describing an unknown secret rejuvenating substance, underlines this aspect of the subject effectively as he describes his favourite rejuvenants.

The first engagement will leave you full of vigour,
The second even stronger than before
Though twelve exquisite beauties, all arranged in scarlet wait your
  onset,

You may enjoy each one according to your fancy,
And, all night through, erect your spear will stand.
In a hundred days, hair and beard will be black once more
In a thousand ways, your body will know its power,
Your teeth will be strong, your eyes more bright.[27]

The Chinese, of course, have from time to time been much pre-occupied with rejuvenation and a remedy still much revered in that country is the incredibly expensive Bird's Nest soup. This has, it will be remembered, "animal and vegetable connections", being made by the sea swallow from seaweed and the spawn of fish, together with, one presumes, certain digestive fluids of the bird itself. One author of a learned book that is mostly concerned with sexual rejuvenation[28] seems to have had personal experience of the famous soup and thinks that its power is due to richness in phosphorous, and warns his readers that "too much can result in a degree of toxic reaction".

Dietetic advice directed towards those who would increase their sexual prowess often falls into the trap of recommending fish for the purpose because it is believed to be rich in phosphorus.

Of course the belief is of great antiquity and Davenport,[9] tells two amusing stories of the alleged power of phosphorus in this matter. In the first a Sultan,

> wishing to ascertain the extent of the continence of the dervishes took two of them into his palace, and during a certain space of time, had them fed on the most succulent food. In this state he gave them two Odalisques of surpassing beauty, but all whose blandishments and allurements proved ineffectual, for the two holy men came forth from the ordeal as pure as the diamond of Bejapore. The Sultan still kept them in his palace ... and caused them to live on a diet equally *recherché* but consisting entirely of fish. Few days later they were again subjected to the combined powers of youth and beauty, but this time nature was too strong. . . .

Elsewhere, Davenport mentions an unhappy incident in which a drake belonging to a chemist fed from a vessel containing phosphorus, and "had not ceased gallanting his females" when he died.

Many authorities, doctors included, have also held this belief. The plain dietetic facts, however, are quite unconvincing. Taken weight for weight, soya flour contains over three times as much phosphorus as caviar, cocoa powder three and a half times as much as lobster, and parmesan cheese nearly six times as much as oysters. Even if we look at fish alone as a source of animal phosphorus, there is little dietetic evidence that the element is involved very much in the various reputations enjoyed by certain species of fish. The well known doggerel,

> Oyster is amorous,
> Lobster is lecherous,
> But shrimps . . .

is somewhat depleted in power when one considers that sardines contain very nearly four times as much phosphorus as shrimps.

It would seem reasonable to suppose that much animal material used in overall rejuvenation is effective merely due to its high protein content and phosphorus or any other elemental derivative has nothing to do with it. Deficiency diseases of all kinds were particularly prevalent in previous centuries when lack of suitable food storage facilities and periodic famine conspired to debilitate, for months on end, large numbers of people. Even in our own times protein-deficiency diseases are productive of syndromes that have symptoms suggestive of senility, which can well be reversed by the intelligent use of protein substances. Dr. John Maddison in his clinic for preventive medicine for older people at Teddington (*see* chapter 11), found that nearly a third of his patients suffered from malnutrition, with protein, vitamin and mineral deficiencies patently obvious. Adequately treated these folk feel, and are, effectively rejuvenated.

Throughout history, however, other inhabitants of the animal world have contributed to ideas on rejuvenation, and it is interesting to observe the unique part that certain species of the *Insecta* have played in this direction. It is rather odd that in this most multifarious form of animal life, which in species alone outnumbers the rest of the animal world and which has adapted itself to live under the most diverse conditions, two specific varieties only are remembered to any extent for their rejuvenating properties. They are the Ant and the common blistering beetles, or Spanish Fly. Of this motley pair one has a potent if unreliable aphrodisiac property, and the other appears to be quite innocuous.

Perhaps typical of recipes for ant-induced rejuvenation is that of John Heyden, who describes himself succinctly as "Gentleman, servant of God and Secretary of Nature". His seventeenth-century *Fortuna Veneris* is worth quoting in full:

Take of pismires or ants, (the biggest having a sourish smell are the best), two handfuls; spirits of wine one gallon: digest them in a glass vessel, close shut, for the space of a month, in which time they will be dissolved into a liquor: then distil them in balneo till all be dry. Then put the same quantity of ants as before: do this three times then aromatise with cinnamon. Note that upon the spirit will float an oil that must be separated. This spirit is excellent to use to stir up the animal spirits. John Casimire Palsgrave of the Rhine and Seyfri of Collen, general against the Turks, did always drink thereof when they went to fight, to increase magnanimity and courage, which it did ever to admiration. This spirit doth also wonderfully irritate them that are sloth to venery.

Formic acid and its salts which occur in ants in considerable quantity were widely exploited as rejuvenating substances well into our century, and perhaps mankind hoped by imbibing remedies made from ants to absorb some of the insect's apparent vigour and indefatigability. However, hopes fell as the pharmacology of these substances was gradually unravelled. On administration by mouth formic acid behaves very much in the same way as does vinegar (acetic acid), which of course it resembles closely chemically. Formate, although metabolized less rapidly than acetate is a relatively innocuous substance, having virtually no demonstrable pharmacological effects. Large quantities of formate are produced regularly within the body and, in man, anything up to 120 milligrams are excreted daily in the urine. Any rejuvenating effects must have come about purely by suggestion.[29]

But if the ant on close investigation appears to have been completely ineffective, the insect world can happily rest on its laurels when the common blistering beetle or Spanish Fly is considered. To be accurate, there is not one but a variety of blistering beetles. As far as European pharmacy is concerned the bright, iridescent golden green or bluish green native of Southern Europe, the

Cantharis vesicatoria, is the usual insect referred to. In America, however, over two hundred species have been described, all of which have a blistering action due to the presence of cantharidic acid.

This substance, contained in the soft parts of the fly, especially its blood, was first isolated by Roviquet in 1810, and for many years Spanish Flies were used both for blistering and rejuvenation. (Blistering or vesication was, until comparatively modern times, a very highly thought of method of medical procedure. Therapeutically it acted in the same way as a liniment or other counter irritant. As such there were many potential uses in medicine, for example in pleurisy, lumbago, neuralgia and rheumatism. Seventeenth- and eighteenth-century medicine abounds in blistering techniques. Some were quite exotic, for example the "flying blister", a series of small blisters applied successively along the course of a nerve, used for instance in sciatica. Often blisters were applied in areas remote from apparent pain. Many of the indications for blistering are the same as those for cupping.)

The Cantharides fly, which incidentally has rarely been found in Southern England during the high summer months, feeds usually upon ash, lilac, privet and jasmine leaves. When present in large numbers they have a powerful and disagreeable smell. Harvesting methods in Spain are simple enough. In the morning and evening, as the temperature falls, the flies become torpid. A cloth is placed under the bush bearing the insects and these are then shaken off and collected. The classical method of killing them is with vinegar or vinegar vapour, after which they are dried and kept in well-stoppered bottles. One of these bottles can be seen in the collection of eighteenth-century drugs at the Pharmaceutical Society's house in Bloomsbury, London, where it forms part of a valuable collection of old drugs presented to the Society by the Royal College of Physicians.

Exactly when cantharides started to be used as an aphrodisiac in England is doubtful. In Continental Europe Spanish Fly preparations were used from the sixteenth century onward and were particularly popular with the French aristocracy. In the latter half of the eighteenth century they were "in much greater vogue than ever before, thanks to Cardinal Richelieu".[30] The Marquis de Sade, of course, gave chocolates laced with Spanish Fly and aniseed, to the four prostitutes during the infamous "Cytherean Morning" of the 27th June, 1772, in Marseilles, so vividly described by Gilbert Lely.[30]

In the *English Dispensatory* of the same year Dr. Quincey [22] describes cantharides under the heading of "diuretics". He mentions also their use as blistering agents and quotes a Dr. Groanvelt's treatise on the use of cantharides preparations internally. This author had been sued for malpractice for using cantharides in this way, and had apparently written the book "in vindication of his own practice". Dr. Quincey states that cantharides "certainly to a strong degree excites lust, and provokes to venereal practices, not by any better abilities which they give, but by stimulating those parts which are the seat or incentives of such desires".

Apparently even in the eighteenth century the dangers of cantharides were realized by physicians, and the *English Dispensatory* quotes the case of a man who, by taking a large dose inwardly, so inflamed himself, that he had almost killed his wife, who declared to the physicians who were sent for next day, that "he that night *septies hortum fodivit:* yet he continued even in distraction with fresh rage until he dy'd delirious".

There is nothing particularly mysterious about the mechanism by which cantharides acts as a sexual stimulant. Cantharidin is readily absorbed from all body surfaces, and the stomach, and is excreted mainly through the kidneys. In the genito-urinary tract it produces reflex stimulation, and, in the male, prolonged erection.

Returning to the notorious Marseilles affair of 1772 previously mentioned, it seems highly likely that both de Sade and his man, Latour, used the cantharides chocolates themselves, otherwise their bizarre sexual exploits would seem impossible on physiological grounds alone. What is more, we are told the sweets were kept "in a bon-bon casket bound in gold", an unnecessarily elaborate container it would seem, if they were only to be presented to common prostitutes. But while the two debauchees probably only took a small dose, de Sade encouraged one of the girls, Marianne, to take seven or eight, and another, Marguerite, an unspecified but large number. The physician, Dr. André Javelier, who gave evidence at the legal proceedings at the Seneschal's Court at Marseilles, when de Sade was prosecuted, describes accurately the symptoms of cantharides poisoning.

"In Marguerite Caste, the poisoning began violently a quarter of an hour after ingestion, taking the form of acute gastric trouble with abundant vomiting of dark matter. . . ." With Marianne the onset of profuse vomiting was delayed some hours. Later signs of lumbar pain and cysto-urethritis occurred in both girls who slowly recovered over a few days. It seems likely that in eighteenth-century France the effects of larger doses of cantharides were not very well known, for neither of the girls, or the examining magistrate, suspected over-dosage with Spanish Fly, and were only worried in case the "stranger" who had outraged them had tried to poison them with arsenic or corrosive sublimate!

Cantharides preparations are rarely used today, either as a blistering preparation or as an aphrodisiac, although official preparations, a Blistering Plaster, a Blistering Liquid and a tincture are still available and could, if required, be prescribed by doctors anywhere.

Before leaving the somewhat strange story of zoological material with reference to rejuvenation, brief reference must be made to the semen in this respect. Havelock Ellis gives a succinct summary of this subject,[6] and apparently the reputation of semen is of great antiquity as a general and sexual rejuvenator. The Aborigines of Australia commonly administer a potion of semen to dying or feeble members of their society, and there is evidence of such belief existing in the folklore of farming districts, where the practice of eating the testes of young lambs when they are castrated is common. In the seventeenth century semen was used as a love philtre, and as a prophylactic in witchcraft. John Hunter, whose devotion to experimental biology apparently persuaded him to taste semen, described it as "warm and spicy", and perhaps this added further to its rejuvenating reputation.

In the nineteenth century a physician writing in a learned medical journal described a case in which the craving for semen as a stimulant in one of his patients was similar to that for alcohol in a dipsomaniac. Strangely, perhaps, Ellis himself, far from being a credulous person, suggested that semen might well be the "physiological aphrodisiac". He also pointed out how science had proved that many substances are easily absorbed by the vaginal epithelium. Semen was thus linked with the development of sexual appetite and maturity of women.

Before completely decrying Havelock Ellis' ideas, based and supported to some extent as they were by Brown-Séquard's work (*see* chapter 8), we should remember that the rather vague substance, *spermin*, studied by various nineteenth-century workers, and that "seemed to be a positive katalysator or accelerator of metabolic processes, exerting a real influence in giving tone to the heart and other muscles, and improving the metabolism of the tissues when all influences of mental suggestion have been excluded", sounds very much like the anabolic steroid substances so much used in modern rejuvenation techniques (*see* chapter 11).

4

Water Cures

It is possible to consider three functions of water in the social history of mankind: social, cleansing and therapeutic. But those who have examined the subject in any detail have often failed to decide the exact use to which water was being put from time to time in early history.

One expert, for instance, in his fascinating book,[31] has drawn attention to the enormous amount of water the Romans used in the fourth century A.D. Some three hundred gallons per head per day is the quantity suggested (in London today we use 51 gallons per head), and St. Paul's Cathedral could fit neatly about six times in the Baths of Caraculla in Rome. But exactly what the Romans expected from their baths either at home or in public remains something of a mystery. One gathers that simple cleanliness was not the prime function. Although the social side of bathing was obviously well catered for, the routine was rather too strict for this to be the first reason for Roman bathing.

There were many local variations on the "bath drill" but it broadly followed this routine. First, it was usual to play a vigorous game, presumably to prepare for what was to follow, and then a warm room or *tepidarium* was entered. Here, perhaps over-hot citizens rested for a while before entering the *apodyterium*, where they undressed and were anointed. Soap was not used and anyone

42

who was particularly dirty received a good rub down with a mixture of oil and sand.

Next came a period in various hot rooms, similar in graduation to those experienced in the modern "turkish" bath, and eventually plenty of water was douched on to the head, first of all hot and then gradually cooler, the method followed atavistically by hairdressers today. After this extensive water treatment Romans usually indulged in a thorough scraping with an ornamental strigil and finished up with a plunge into the cold water of the *frigidarium*.

To what extent the Romans expected these elaborate bathing arrangements to improve their health we do not know. But there seems no doubt at all that the higher up the social scale the greater was the devotion to the Bath, until the point was reached when certain Emperors bathed up to eight times a day. It is difficult to equate this with an excessive desire for cleanliness or sociability however. The custom of "mixed" bathing in the Roman baths with all the suggestion of promiscuity implied by those who have written on this topic certainly suggests that Roman bathers eventually tended to look upon the Baths as places where flagging sexual energies might be stimulated, and so rejuvenation becomes linked with public bathing.

It may be argued that in their support of rejuvenation by water the Romans were echoing ideas expressed in the ancient literary language of India some thousand years or more previously. Unfortunately the history of Sanskrit literature labours under the disadvantage of an almost total absence of any fixed chronology. But modern experts feel that the sacred canon of the Rig-Veda was expressed at about 1000 B.C. The Rig-Veda (Knowledge or Love of praise), tells of Cyavana the Saint being rejuvenated by two physician-gods. The methodology was simple for he was merely thrown into a miraculous river.

The Vedic physicians of the Gods, the Nâsatyas, apparently knew well of water's rejuvenating properties for they themselves were elevated to the status of gods by the rejuvenation of a certain elderly husband of Sukanyâ, a beautiful woman. Watching her bathing one day they called to her saying:

"O woman of delicious limbs, why did thy father bestow thee on such an old man, on the edge of the grave. Thou art as radiant as summer lightning, we have seen none like thee even in heaven. Even without any ornament thou art an embellishment to the whole forest. How much more beautiful wouldst thou be in rich robes and splendid jewels! Abandon thine ancient husband and choose one of us, for youth does not endure". She replied that she could not do this due to her wifely devotion. Sportingly, perhaps, or suspecting that the young wife felt bound to an age-ing man for reasons of responsibility rather than love, the physi-cians suggested rejuvenating him. Husband and wife agreed and he bathed in the lake alongside the Nâsatyas and "all three emerged young and radiant". Sukanyâ had difficulty picking out her husband, so alike did the three men appear in their youthful-ness, but eventually she chose the right man, who, delighted with his youth and the fidelity of his wife, persuaded the God Indra to include the twin Nâsatyas among the Gods.[32]

Other Hindu legends stress the importance of water in reju-venation. The eagle which plunged into a fountain and was re-juvenated reappears in Mesopotamian mythology and it may be the bird referred to in the 103rd Psalm: "who satisfieth thy mouth with good things, so that thy youth is renewed like the eagle's".

Other ancient civilizations showed a preference for water in the service of rejuvenation. For instance the Japanese believed in the fountain lore of Kiku-Jido (Chrysanthemum Boy), and how the petals of his flowers dipped in saki brought blessings of long life and health.[33]

In the Middle Ages it is possible to trace, with a reasonable degree of certainty, the spread to Europe of the idea that water was a rejuvenating substance, through certain aspects of ecclesias-tical history. Although its founder, the Christian theologian Nestorius, had died a condemned heretic by the middle of the fifth century, a Nestorian church grew up by the beginning of the sixth century under the protection of the Rulers of Persia. Originally formed by east Syrian and Persian Christians, it sur-vived the subsequent Arab conquerors, who treated the Nestorians tolerantly, and for some eight hundred years the Nestorian

Church flourished. It embraced and attracted learned philosophers and theologians and physicians, and its missionary expansion eventually interacted with the cultures of India and China. As well as introducing its own brand of Christianity into these countries the Nestorians were probably also influenced by Eastern folklore and mythology. As such they seem to have injected into Eastern life much of the East's folklore and myth, including ideas about rejuvenation through bathing.

One such example comes to light in the story of Prester John, the phantom King of the Orient. The idea was widespread that there was an actual Christian King and conqueror of enormous power and significance hidden somewhere in Europe from the end of the twelfth century till well into the fourteenth. The earliest mention of such a person is in the chronicle of Otho, Bishop of Freising in Bavaria. During the year 1145 while the bishop was at the Papal Court he heard from the bishop of Gabala all about one John, king and priest who "dwelt in the extreme Orient beyond Persia and Armenia, who was, with his people, a Christian but Nestorian". He had battled against the Persian hordes and was advancing to fight, in aid of the church, at Jerusalem, but had been halted at the Tigris which had proved impossible to ford.

In support of Bishop Otho's chronicle is a letter, copies of which flooded Europe some twenty years later. Around one hundred manuscripts have been described, and eight are in the possession of the British Museum.[34] The contents of these letters made a fantastic impression on the medieval mind.

Presbyter or Prester John was a decidely extravagent character. Describing himself the "greatest monarch under heaven" he claimed to rule over seventy-two kings, the lands of whom extended over "the three Indies, including that Further India where lay the body of St. Thomas" and "the ruins of Babylon and the Tower of Babel".

Explaining his self-effacing title, for Presbyter really means Elder, he wrote that this was merely evidence of his humility. And in any case what grand title could effectively describe a ruler so elevated as to be waited on at table by a "Primate and a King, whose butler was an archbishop and a King, whose chamberlain was a bishop and a King, whose master of the horse was an abbot and a King".[35] The kingdom of such a potentate was, of course, filled with much more than ordinary things. There were pebbles that gave sight, or alternatively rendered the possessor invisible, a subterranean stream whose sands were made of gems. A creature called salamander which, wrapped in an incombustible envelope, lived on fire, and there were ants which dug up gold. Understandably there were no poor in these dominions. Neither were there criminals, flatterers, liars or dissenters, partly perhaps because of a marvellous mirror erected on a splendid many-tiered platform in which the Presbyter could see everything that went on in his whole domain and presumably detect the potential enemy of society at an early stage. Not the least of the wonders of Prester John's kingdom was, however, the Fountain of Youth.

Of this, all that was necessary was to "Taste thrice daily on a fasting stomach for three years, three months and three hours" to live and remain youthful for "three hundred years, three months, three weeks, three days and three hours". Concerning the exact location of the fountain the Presbyter remained unexpectedly reticent and only tells us that it was "less than three days' journey from the river of Paradise" (the Ganges). Others put it in the mainland of India, or at Adam's Park in Ceylon, the site from which Buddha is believed to have ascended into heaven.

Several suggestions have been put forward by historians to explain the Prester John legend, and the curious letter which was thought of seriously enough to be officially replied to by Pope Alexander III in 1177. This reply, which is in the Paris National Library, was to have been delivered to Prester John by the Pope's son, Philip the Physician. It has been suggested that Prester John was Gur Khan of Black Cathay or perhaps the Georgian Prince John Orbelian, a famous generalissimo under several kings of Georgia of that age. Another theory suggested he was the Christian King of Abyssinia, and it was to the latter that Pope Alexander III addressed his memorable letter. From the fourteenth century onwards Prester John was presumed to have his mythical kingdom in Abyssinia.

But by now the legend of the Fountain of Youth was well established in Europe. As such it was referred to in the art and literature of the age in many ways. The twelfth-century poem *Roman d'Alexandre* gives a falsely romantic account of the bestial crimes against humanity committed by Alexander the Great. But in it it is possible to read how the insatiable warrior, whose thirst for blood was only exceeded apparently by that he had for wine, discovered "a fountain surrounded by evergreens in a refulgent landscape: the magic waters gush from the mouth of an old gelder lion into a basin in a crystal pavilion: Alexander and fifty-six of his men drank deeply there and were rejuvenated, their complexions being restored to the age of thirty". When one considers that Alexander the Great was only thirty-three when he died after a prodigious drinking bout and carousal, it seems likely that such rejuvenation as he received at the Fountain of Youth was rather minimal.

Many European artists took the Fountain of Youth together with the joys of bathing as themes for painting. Lucas Cranach was one of the representative painters of Germany during the Reformation. He had a curious career, even for a painter at this time, holding at one time the monopoly of the sale of medicine at Wittenberg as well as a printer's patent with exclusive privileges as to copyright in Bibles. Friend or confidant of Luther, who incidentally used his printing presses, most of Cranach's paintings are of conventional subjects, hunting scenes, madonnas, religious and mythological subjects featuring recurrently in his repertoire. A painting of the fountain of youth in a style vaguely reminiscent of Breugel, however, gives an interesting insight into current ideas on this interesting subject.

The centre of the picture shows a square "swimming pool" type of bath of perhaps 200 by 100 foot dimensions. Two steps run around the edge to facilitate entry into the pool. At one end of the pool is a twenty-foot-high fountain which introduces the water. About twenty people of mixed sex are bathing naked. On the left-hand side of the picture the old and the infirm are brought on horseback, by carriage, wheelbarrow, stretcher or on pick-a-back. They undress on the edge and plunge in. On the right-hand side of the pool they are seen leaving rejuvenated. Disappearing into nearby changing tents they finally leave, grandly attired, to take their places at a tremendous alfresco picnic in the nearby countryside.

A prevalent belief in Spain in the early sixteenth century was that a miraculous spring existed in the New World on an island originally called Bimimi. Legend had it that the glittering wings of an angel who drank from the spring each day, fell into the water and imbued it with the power to rejuvenate and beautify. Juan Ponce de Leon, born of an ancient Spanish family, ultimately obtained a patent from King Ferdinand to discover and explore this much-sought-after island.

Ferdinand V goes down in history as a particularly ungracious monarch who broke his promises and openly bragged of his deceit. Although over sixty at the time when he grudgingly allowed the Ponce de Leon to go and seek Bimimi he was not interested in rejuvenation. What is more he apparently had little time for explorers, stating bluntly that "all that can now be discovered is very easy to discover". The King, however, was always keen on treasure. The patent granted to the Ponce allowed him to retain one-tenth of the revenue that might accrue from his exploration for twelve years, making no specific mention of springs or fountains of youth.

The Ponce de Leon and his party of explorers eventually set out from Spain, and on 27th March, 1513, under the guidance of Columbus' navigator, Anton de Alaminos, sighted what was believed to be the beautiful island they were seeking. As it was Easter Sunday they named it Florida (Pascua Florida). Although the Ponce de Leon, it is said, became disenchanted with the idea of a fountain of youth, there is every likelihood he discovered some of the famous springs of Florida, notably the WaKulla, the Manatee spring and the Silver spring, that fascinated many later visitors.

Many of these springs of Florida have been commercialized in the twentieth century, for example, the Ponce de Leon Springs in St. Augustine, close to where the Ponce and his party originally landed. A nineteenth-century writer describes the Silver spring,[36]

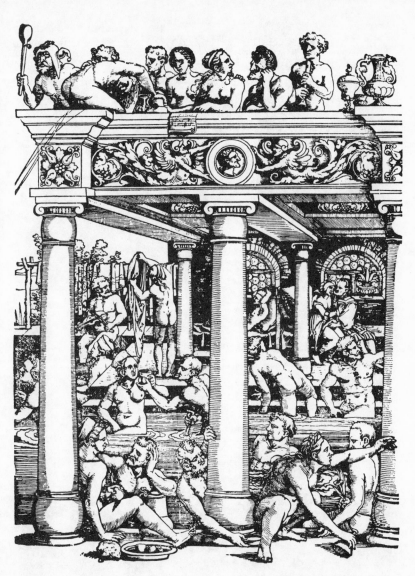

This "Fountain of Youth" indicates the frivolity as well as the
sexuality prevalent at such places

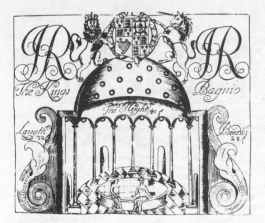

Upon the great Encouragement I received from the Kings Moſt Excellent Majeſty ; from His late Majeſty of Ever Bleſſed Memory ; from the Nobility and Gentry, and from many Eminent Phyſicians and others of great Learning and Travell, I Erected a Bagnio in *Long-Acre*, known by the Name of the *King's-Bagnio* ; and by His Majeſty, the Nobility and Gentry highly Approved.

And by Experience of Thouſands, found to be of great Uſe and Benefit for all Man-kind ; not only to ſuch as are in perfect Health, to continue it and prevent Diſtempers, but of wonderful and ſure Relief, to all Aged, Weak, and Conſumptive Perſons of both Sex, and to all in General, who are afflicted with any Chronical Diſeaſes ; Bed-rid Perſons, and ſuch as by Rheumatiſms Ach, &c. have had no Uſe of their Limbs, have been Reſtored to Admiration. Now for that, the conſtant Price hath hitherto been Five Shillings and Sixpence.

That now, all manner of Perſons may receive ſo great a Benefit, with leſs Charge. I have thought fit, notwithſtanding the great Expence of Building, and daily Charge attending it to retrench the Prizes, and do hereby declare, that from, and after the Date herof, That if two come together in Company, they ſhall pay but Eight Shillings ; if three, but Eleven Shillings ; that if one ſingle Perſon comes three times in 14 Days, he ſhall have the like Advantage.

Tueſdays, and *Fridays* for Women, and the other Days for Men.

From the King's-Bagnio,
March, 25. 1686.

Sir *William Jennens* Kt.
Sworn Servant to His
Majeſty for the *Bagnio.*

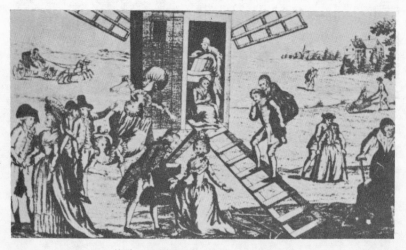

"The Windmill of Rejuvenation"

and from his writings one can capture some of the mystery that gave the legend of Springs of Youth so much of their allure:

> In December 1856 I had opportunity to examine it [the Silver Spring], with the aid of special instruments. To be appreciated in its full beauty, it should be approached from the Ocklewaha. For more than a week I had been tediously ascending this river in a pole barge, wearied by the monotony of the dark and gloomy forests that every-where shade its inky stream, when one bright morning a short turn brought us into the pellucid waters of the Silver Spring Run. A few vigorous strokes and we had left the cypress swamps and emerged in broad, level savannas.

He goes on to mention the tropical vegetation, innumerable flowers and splendid local bird life which gave a particularly idyllic setting to the spring, and was particularly impressed with "the subaqueous landscape", in which enormous trout and catfish hovered over glorious aquatic plants. The basin of the spring which was described as elliptical in form, (diameter 150 yards, conjugate 100 yards), was forty-one feet deep.

> When the sunbeams fall full on the water, by a familiar optical delu-sion, it seems to a spectator . . . that the bottom and sides of the basin are elevated, and over the whole, over the frowning crags, the snow white shells, the long sedge, and the moving aquatic tribes, the decomposed light flings its rainbow hues, and all things float in a sea of colours, magnificent and impressive beyond description. What wonder that the untaught children of nature spread the fame of this marvellous fountain to far distant climes, and under the stereoscopic power of time and distance come to regard it as the life-giving stream, whose magic waters washed away the calamities of age, and the pains of disease, round whose fortunate shores youths and maidens ever sported eternally young and eternally joyous.

The author of these words gives no further account of whether the Silver Spring was actually being used by nineteenth-century Americans, but we do know that hydrotherapy was established in several places in America by this time. One lightly written book [37] gives an interesting enough account of "Life, Love and Death at the Waters", to be included in the bibliography of the subject.

As we have seen, any ideas with reference to the rejuvenating properties of water that flourished in the New World originated from Europe. But exactly how much therapeutic effect upon this score was expected or obtained from bathing in or drinking "the waters" during the period between the Middle Ages and the nineteenth century remains in doubt. Much of the confusion probably arises because other factors relative to religious feeling, social intercourse and public or private pleasure have clouded the picture.

From the very beginning the fathers of the Church were against public bathing, therapeutic or otherwise. "Women will scarce strip naked before their husbands, effecting a plausible pretence of modesty, but any others who wish, may see them at home, shut up in their own baths, for they are not ashamed to strip before spectators, as if exposing their persons for sale. The baths are opened promiscuously to women: and there they strip for licentious indulgence, (for, from looking, men get to loving), as if their modesty had been washed away in the bath."[38]

This expressed sentiment was echoed by churchmen throughout the Middle Ages and well on into modern times. Pope Adrian I, however, mitigated these rather strict censures when he recommended his parochial clergy to visit the baths in grand procession every Thursday.

From the purely social point of view, of course, the popularity of bathing fluctuated through the centuries, and there is a point of contact here between the development of the various spas and the presence throughout the civilized world of holy springs and wells. Here "men prayed first and were healed afterwards. How they were healed was a mystery: but the cure, it was thought, came from the saint, not the water. After the Reformation, when the saints were no longer allowed to have mysteries, the holy wells became wishing wells".[39]

Another change, however, took place as a result of this attitude, for some of the faith that mankind previously maintained for saintly or religious cures gradually became grafted on to the doctors. And so "the waters" either imbibed or bottled provided in a way a new magic for mankind. That this had scientific rather than religious roots made it no less seductive. It is impossible, as

previously stated, to separate the social, cleansing and thereapeu-
tic properties of water in any hard and fast way. Nevertheless the
great boom in hydrotherapy as such coincided with the end of
the first quarter of the nineteenth century, when for the first time
it was possible to analyse water scientifically, and for medical
men to question seriously what water would do as far as rejuvenation was concerned.

Always there had been doctors who were enthusiastic on the
subject. Dr. Lodwick Rowzee, who practised at Ashford in
Kent, was quite precise when he recommended Tunbridge water
for enlivening "the nobler parts of the body and spirits", producing
"a sweet balsamick, spiritous and sanguinous temperament:
which naturally incites men and women to amorous emotions
and titillations" and "enabling them to procreation".[41]

Dr. Rowzee believed in the aphorism that it is impossible to
have too much of a good thing and recommended his patients to
drink three hundred ounces of water during the morning.
Happily, perhaps, he enjoined them also to exercise, "use their
legges" and "stirre them up and down". After quaffing over
eighteen pints of Tunbridge water they would scarcely have been
able to do otherwise.

As might be expected, other doctors gave contrary advice.
For instance, Dr. Diederick Wessel Linden, whose Treatise on
the *Origin, Nature and Virtues of Chalybeat waters, and Natural
Hot Baths*, was published in 1748, and who prefaced his work with
several sycophantic poems composed by his friends living at
smart London addresses, could not recommend the waters for
these purposes. His reasons are interesting, throwing as they do
some light on eighteenth-century medicine. Mineral waters were
contra-indicated in those over sixty, because they "dispose by
their native, inherent astringency and dry quality, the elementary
particles to cohesion". This, Dr. Linden felt, accelerated the
ageing processes which he had already noted, and tended to
diminish the number, size and elasticity of the blood vessels in the
body.

Nevertheless the spas and hydrotherapeutic establishments definitely seemed to cater especially for the aged and those who

sought to find lost youth. Many semi-humorous books were written in the middle of the nineteenth century about spa life. Almost
always the elderly patient or "guest" is described therein. One [40]
told of "an inmate of Marienberg . . . a lady who numbered nearly
fourscore years", undergoing a course of hydropathy. She was
"the widow of one who was second to none in the branch of
medical science which he followed, and to which he contributed
some of the most valuable and scientific works". The author felt
that on the whole she did not respond well to treatment, but
wisely remarked, "the ills of old age are not easily removed".[41]

Another interesting book gives us unique insight into an establishment at Malvern, run by Dr. James Wilson.[42] Its author is an
intelligent man with fine powers of observation and description.
By profession a lithographer to Queen Victoria and Prince Albert,
he had been dogged by a variety of ailments, the description of
which defies retrospective diagnosis even today. Obviously well
off, living in his house on the banks of London's Regent's Canal,
he ran more or less the whole gauntlet of Victorian therapeutics,
including the blue pill and dose system, the morning draught,
calomel, and a daily dose of taraxocum, (a preparation made from
the dried roots and rhizome of the dandelion). Not dismayed he
moved on to galvanism and although this ameliorated his symptoms, which at the time were neuralgic pains followed by the
sensation that he had a "cork leg", he soon relapsed and was enjoined to try the water cure "as a duty" by his intimate friend, Sir
E. Bulwer Lytton.

Space prevents any further elaboration of the details of the cure,
which was preceded by a trip on the new Birmingham Railway
and a chance encounter with a coachman who somewhat subdued the patient's enthusiasm by remarking that if he "kept good
hours and lived regularly" he would "do just as well without Dr.
Wilson". Suffice it to say that by Dr. Wilson he was cured and
was so enthusiastic that he felt it incumbent upon him to try to
set up a hydropathic club in London, à la Malvern. At Malvern
there were clearly many whose aim was rejuvenation. One was
"a broken down swell" who was "sadly used up" when Dr.
Wilson took him on as a patient. Under a rigorous regime of

hydropathy, together with dietary restriction to "nine ounces of solid food in the day and as much water as he can drink" the "poor fellow" rallied.

Eventually recovery was complete and although it came as something of a shock to find that the "broken down swell" was not a lord but "a respectable hairdresser from a manufacturing town", it was obviously pleasant to see him so nicely rejuvenated.

References in Victorian books on sexual rejuvenation are not all that easy to find, probably due to contemporary rigour, and yet a typical case is described at the Water Cure in Malvern.

"A very worthy couple, past the meridian of life who had been married eighteen years, had no children. They had lived an artificial life of much gaiety, and had deemed it necessary to have a physician in close attendance for ten or twelve years." Eventually they were persuaded to take the water cure and soon a baby was expected.

It is impossible to leave any account of nineteenth-century hydropathy and its relationship to rejuvenation without paying tribute to a curious practitioner of the art, Vincent Priessnitz. Priessnitz was a semi-literate Silesian peasant who stumbled across hydrotherapy in a curious way. When he was a boy of thirteen he sustained a sprained wrist and cured it by binding up his arm with wet bandages. Three years later he had more trouble when a riding accident fractured some of his ribs and knocked out his front teeth. There is still no really effective way of treating fractured ribs other than by a simple strapping that is thought to immobilize and support the affected part. In the middle of the nineteenth century, not surprisingly, Priessnitz's doctors offered no specific advice, and so the patient decided once again to try water. The fact that he was free of symptoms a year later he put down to the water cure, not nature, and the world's most famous hydrotherapist was born.

It is said that Priessnitz started his water healing free of charge for neighbours, and he cured many people "given up by doctors". Eventually, however, Priessnitz was in business in a big way, and by 1843 he had over fifteen hundred patients and was said to have a bank balance of £50,000.

Priessnitz was an odd man "built with broad shoulders, without any tendency to fat, five feet eight inches in height, with an excellent phrenological development: having his front teeth knocked out, appearing a larger man at a distance than he is found to be when you are closer".[43] He tended to make remarks, on the spur of the moment, that could not under any circumstances have gone down well with his patients. For instance, when a patient died during treatment, he opined that "he had too short a neck for a long life". Nevertheless, Priessnitz flourished and in his heyday catered almost exclusively for rich Germans hoping to regain the joys of lost youth. That they could be invalids in the strict sense of the word, would seem to be ruled out by the diet provided by Priessnitz for his patients:

> The food at Graefenberg is served in the German fashion of abundance and greasy cookery. The patients are allowed, and even encouraged, to eat abundantly of roast meats, fish, green vegetables, cheese and other preparations of milk and fruits. . . . The patients of Priessnitz, acting under his advice, may be said to devour rather than eat, and they gradually acquire a habit in this respect that is difficult to eradicate. No attempt is made at modification of regimen adapted to different ages, sexes, habits and morbid affections.[44]

Further evidence that patients at Graefenberg were by and large perfectly fit people in search of some form of physical stimulation, rather than treatment in the medical sense, is suggested by the rigour of the Priessnitz regime. The water from the spring ran out at anything between forty-three and fifty-two degrees Fahrenheit, and with this icy fluid patients were douched, sprinkled or wrapped up in sheets and bathed. Constitutionally they must have been extremely sound to have withstood the "treatment".

Graefenberg-type hydropathic establishments were popular all over England in the nineteenth century. A veteran water doctor of the time, whose practice was typical of many of his colleagues, was Edward Johnson, M.D., of Malvern, who wrote a book [43] on the subject, assisted by his sons, Drs. Walter and Haward Johnson. The former was at one time medical tutor at Guy's Hospital. Johnson used all the standard Priessnitz techniques, believing that hydropathic treatment could cure all ills, and his enthusiasm knew no bounds. What is more he attempted to establish a *rationale* for water treatments:

> It does not deal with mere symptoms. It goes at once to the root of the matter. It deals with principles and causes. It does not tinker with the human body and mend it with patches. It takes a great and general and comprehensive view of disease and its causes. . . . It claims to be sensible, rational and in harmony with the known laws which regulate and govern life, health and disease. . . . I have shown that the pores of the skin, if joined end to end, would form a tube twenty-eight miles in length. Surely there can be no difficulty in believing that if this tube be obstructed and the matters which it is intended to carry out of the blood be left in it, while the matters which it is intended to convey into the blood be kept out of it,— surely, I say, there can be no difficulty in believing that a very unhealthy and wrong state of the blood must be the necessary result. And it must surely be apparent that any treatment which has the power of restoring or augmenting the function of this stupendous secreting tube, must be capable of exercising a beneficial influence on health, and through this means alone, of curing many diseases. How plain and common sense this appears. How rational! How intelligible!

Eventually there seems to have been something like a schism in the medical profession, leading to the establishment dividing into "drug doctors" and "water doctors", although judging by medical students' examination papers published in the *Lancet*, in 1840, a sound knowledge of the principles of hydrotherapy was highly necessary for all doctors who wanted to pass their examinations.

Eventually the whole subject of hydrotherapy became important enough to need its own textbooks. Typical of many was one published in 1896 described as an authority on balneo-therapeutic management as well as of spas and hydros.[46] Of course there was little specific medical therapy available at the turn of the century. And so even quite eminent medical men can be excused for convincing themselves that hydrotherapy could cure almost any disease. The water cure flourished and widened its therapeutic spectrum even further. The book mentioned had reached its third edition by 1907 and its main author was now Sir Hermann Weber.

The rejuvenating qualities of "the waters" were not forgotten, and the Spas of Ems and Gastein were recommended for old age and premature senility, having been the favourite of Kaiser Wilhelm I, who lived to be ninety-one, and that of Cannes by Lord Brougham who survived to be ninety years old. By now, of course, the spas were much more involved with the broad principles of physiotherapy and less was heard of drinking the waters and hydrotherapy generally.

Hydrotherapy seems to have died a natural death in Great Britain and there seems no doubt that its demise was accelerated by the introduction of the National Health Service in 1949. A cyclostyled letter of introduction to one of Britain's few remaining centres of hydrotherapy informed patients that "A National Health prescription will be made out which is to be taken to the Royal Baths". A psychological shiver goes down the spine at the very thought of it. Then, of course, the "waters" themselves can be obtained incredibly cheaply. Chalybeate, Crescent saline, or Kissingen (hot, cold or aerated), are a mere sixpence a glass, and the public, whether they have rejuvenation or anything else in mind, are persuaded privately that something so inexpensive cannot possibly be any good. Calls for Malvern or Vichy water are now heard only in relation to the cocktail bar and not the pump room.

In West Germany, however, the spa, although admittedly far removed from the eccentric principles of Father Graefenberg, still holds tremendous sway. A rejuvenating holiday where everyone gets a taste of long-lost youth is still well to the fore in the German mind. A contemporary survey lists as many as 144 spas, thirty hydropathic spas and twenty-five climato-therapeutic resorts, at which water plays a prominent part. But alongside hydrotherapy there is a beautiful countryside, swimming pools, golf and tennis and wide cultural interests to stimulate patients as well. Enough in all probability to make one feel and maybe look, at the end of the "treatment", somewhat rejuvenated by the power of water.

5

Fringe Rejuvenation Methods

The fact that an idea is basically commercial rather than altruistic or even scientific makes it no less worthy of study. Indeed, sometimes in their basic urge to earn an easy living at the expense of a gullible and misinformed public, quacks have made worthwhile contributions to the history of science.[47] Although quackery, as an expression of mankind's exploitation of his ill-informed brothers, is probably as old as civilization itself, until firm foundations begin to be laid in medical science it is unprofitable to examine the subject in any detail.

Such a state of affairs certainly obtained at the close of the sixteenth century in England and an early example of a medical man who catered for quack rejuvenation was Francis Anthony. Having gained an M.A. at Cambridge, he set up medical practice in London, but omitted to obtain a licence from the College of Physicians. Thus he was soon arraigned before the President and Censors of the College of Physicians who found him "weak and ignorant" in "several parts of physic". Anthony must have faced his examiners when they were in a very testy mood for they fined him £20 and threw him into prison, from whence he was not released until two years later in 1602.[48]

The reason for the severe punishment (many less qualified colleagues escaped with a warning and a polite invitation to appear before the censors again), may well have been because Anthony passed himself off as a rejuvenator rather than an orthodox physician. In all probability he was an embarrassment to the small number of doctors practising in London at this time, due to the success of his prescription, Aurum Potabile.

The incorruptibility of gold to corrosion was possibly the reason for a wide belief, in the sixteenth and seventeenth century, that medicines containing gold acted as rejuvenants. Anthony made no bones about his recipe for this elixir of life, and eventually published a small pamphlet giving full details.[49] The process consisted of making a "menstruum" of tin oxide which was "digested" in red wine and vinegar. Then this was allowed to react on powdered gold (at £3 13s. 4d. an ounce), which had been previously heated up with salt. A solution of stearate of gold was eventually prepared, a substance of some toxicity. At least one of Anthony's patients, a "Reverend Devine", complained on his deathbed that his fate was due to Aurum Potabile. Solutions of gold salts can have no rejuvenating effect, and yet such "Quintessences of Gold", as they were often called, remained popular with quacks and their patients for many a year.

Similarly, some rejuvenation quacks at this time trafficked in "counterfeit" unicorn's horn, actually made of rhinoceros horn. Unicorn's horn was a favoured ingredient of many a seventeenth-century physician's prescription.

Another idea that came to light in the middle of the seventeenth century was to use Orvietan as a rejuvenant. Orvietan, initially claimed to be a universal antidote against poison, was named after Orvieto in Italy, from whence it was thought to hail. A small step forward in thought brings the theory that by driving out poison, the body becomes rejuvenated, *pari passu*.

Typical of the hawkers of this chicanery was Cornelius Tilburg (or Tilbourne), who called himself, *à la mode*, a High German Doctor and Physician, Oculist, Chirurgeon and Rupture Master. Tilburg seems to have been an extraordinary man and probably Charles II and later King William and Queen Mary consulted him for he claimed that these monarchs gave him a special licence to practise physic and dispense his "excellent and never-failing remedies".

Another member of the Tilburg family carried on the rejuvenation cures when Cornelius retired. This James Tilburg, as well as claiming to cure the French pox, a disease he described as being due to an "anchoring in a strange harbour", also advertised that he could rejuvenate as well as his predecessor. "He helps them that have lost their nature and cherishes up the saddened spirits of a married man by what occasion so ever they have lost it, and does quicken them again as a Rose that hath received the summer's dew."[50]

The principle of polypharmacy, so dear to the seventeenth-century mind, exemplified *par excellence* in the multifarious mithridate and theriac, was also evoked by those whose ambitions were more attuned to a profitable financial exercise than any scientific idea. Theriac, based on Venice Treacle and quite respectably housed in the *Pharmacopaea* of the Royal College of Physicians of London as late as 1724, contained sixty-two ingredients. An Italian quack named Salvator Winter, who practised from his house at the "Sign of St. Paul's Head", New King Street, Covent Garden in London, advertised that his *Elixir Vitae* contained an equal number of ingredients. Winter, who claimed to be eighty-nine years old, yet "by the Blessing of God finds himself in health as strong as anyone of fifty", maintained that he carried a bottle of his "sovereign remedy" with him night and day, taking a dose whenever he felt the need of it. Like many quacks Winter believed firmly in the power of the testimonial and blatantly boasted of having one from Sir Kenhelm Digby.

Not all quacks, however, leant on orthodox medical practice to support their wares. Ben Willmore, a contemporary of Salvator Winter, who practised mostly at Tower Hill, still an area of London where the gullible can easily be relieved of their coin, relied purely on showmanship to promote his trade. Dressed in a scarlet coat, braided with gold and wearing a feathered cocked hat, he harangued the crowd with talk of "The Old Made Young". In a bill printed in 1680 he claimed, "I will not pretend that I have made my great Restorer cure any distemper, excepting one, and such a one, as I believe was never helped by any medicine but this, that is to say in Love Affairs both in Old Men and

Women". The Restorer made, he alleged, those of "three or four score as youthful as those of twenty or thirty years old".

A method of boosting sales of a rejuvenant that has hardly been bettered was exploited nicely by another well known seventeenth-century quack, Moses Stringer. He addressed himself in what purported to be private letters written to Dr. Woodrofe, Master of Worcester College, Oxford:

> Sir, Since I had the honour of your Instructions in the University concerning physick and chemistry, I have in a particular manner, apply'd myself to the study of those sciences. I have considered the nature of Humane Bodies and consulted the History of the Ancients, tho' yet, what Paracelsus reports concerning the force of medicines in Recovering Old Age, affects me very much.

> That Learned Chymist made his first experiment upon a Hen, so very old that nobody would kill it, either out of a sense of profit or good nature. He mingled some of his medicine, which he called Renovating Quintessence, with a quantity of Barley and gave it to the Hen, fifteen days together. The effects were wonderful, and the Hen recovered Youth and New Feathers, and what is still more surprising, Laid Eggs and Hatcht chickens as if she had lost a dozen years of her age.

> But this small experiment in Animals did not content the inquisitions of that Scrutinous Chymist, who turned his skill to the relief of mankind. An ancient woman who kept house for him, with the consequences of Old Age, was upon the very margin of Death. He gave her the same medicine fifteen days together, as that prescribed to his feathered patient, and with similar success. She recovered her Health, Youth, Hair and Teeth again. Her complexion looked florid and vigorous and Nature exerted itself as it generally does in Young Women.

> Reflecting upon these Cures, and the probity and candour of the Physician from when they proceeded, I thought such a remedy might be formed as might renew youth very much and help Old Age.

> Some years since, with considerable cost and pains, I had the good fortune to find out two medicines of general use, the "Elixir Febrifugum Martis" and "Salt of Lymons", but finding, (th' the cures effected by them were surprising), yet they did not extend to renew Age so much as I could have wish't, I therefore, a second time, endeavoured and I hope have found, a Medicine which very much lessens the Infirmities of Age, renders Nature vigorous and stretches the Span of Human Life as far as Heaven Permits.

It is difficult to equate anything very much of Stringer's bill with writings of Paracelsus on Rejuvenation which were wildly vague anyhow. His readers, however, were unlikely to check the source literature and the sales technique employed probably sold gallons of Elixir Renovans which he marketed from a house at Puddle Dock, Blackfriars, a site close by the home of the Hall of the Worshipful Society of Apothecaries of London.

Other techniques of the seventeenth-century rejuvenators, taking advantage of every facet of medical abandonment liable to be experienced by the unfortunate patient, can be seen in the activities of later contemporary operators. The "given up by doctors" routine, exploited so successfully in the United States in modern times, finds early expression in a handbill of Stringer's in which he tells of a wretched patient, once a slave in Algiers, and prematurely old and worn out at fifty-five, who was rejuvenated by him so successfully that he was "absolutely recovered plump and fit" by a course of Elixir Renovans—this after the doctors of St. Thomas's Hospital had been unable to help him despite a whole year's treatment.

Another harbinger of what was to be successful quack rejuvenation technique in later times also has its origins in the seventeenth century. Cognisant, as most intelligent men were, of the benefits of "taking the waters" in the seventeenth century (*see* chapter 4), John Coniers, an apothecary of Shoe Lane, was probably the first to light upon the happy idea of bottling an essence that would convert, he claimed, ordinary waters into medicated spring water. "Any soft spring water mixt with a little thereof, becomes in nature a True Tunbridge Water of great use to those desirous to be spared ye journey to ye Wells", a handbill proudly told his patients.

The eighteenth century, broadly speaking, followed the general tenor of the previous hundred years as far as rejuvenation quackery was concerned. The only really notable change was the change in status of some of the quacks in question. Most of the early rejuvenators were little better than travelling salesmen who hawked their wares at street corners and market places, taking advantage of a crowd or conglomeration of potential customers whenever the occasion presented itself. In the eighteenth century, however, quack rejuvenators became quite important people. Often they were supported by the attention of nobility and frequently they practised from quite elaborate establishments.

Typical of many, but perhaps more successful than most of his brethren was the famous James Graham (1745–94), whose practice of rejuvenation quackery was at its peak in London in the 1780s. Like many of his brethren Graham entered rejuvenation quackery as a side line. The full story of James Graham, Master Quack, has been told elsewhere,[41] but a few highlights of his career as a rejuvenator are not out of place.

As early as 1777 Graham was specializing in electrical treatments for various unspecified diseases. He travelled extensively in his early days in the British Isles, France and America, and claimed to have met and talked to the great Benjamin Franklin on both sides of the Atlantic.

In the year 1780 he seemed to crystallize his wide experience of quack practice and as a result eventually opened his impressive Temple of Health in an elegant ten-roomed Adam house in Adelphi Terrace, London. To make quite sure it was easily distinguished, and to give his clientele an idea of what he was providing, Graham had an enormous golden star fixed on to the front of the house, and the words *Templum Aesculapia Sacrum* emblazoned over the porch. Contemporary sources give evidence that Graham's initial venture was a great success. Representative of his patients was Henry Angelo, one time fencing master to the Court of George IV who wrote, "I remember the carriages drawing up next to the door of this modern Paphos, with crowds of gaping sparks on either side, to discover who were the visitors, but the ladies' faces were covered, all going incognito".[51]

Once inside the Temple, Graham's patients found themselves in lavishly decorated rooms. The largest was used as a lecture hall. Here Graham gave his famous addresses, and told his audience what could be expected if his medicines were taken and his general principles followed. He also provided a little amusement, by means of simple electrical experiments and finally showed off scantily-clothed girls, referred to as Goddesses of Health. His clientele were then advised that they could easily obtain similar grace and beauty if only they followed the Graham method.

Elsewhere in the house Graham prepared and made his various medicines. Originally there were twelve of these.

1. *The Imperial Pill*, "absolutely infallible for all bilious, gouty and rheumatic complaints"
2. *Anti-scorbutic Essence*, "purifier of the blood and humours"
3. *Vegetable Balsam*, "for cooling and cleaning every outward malady"
4. *Pearl Essence*, "for healing all ulcers, cankers, cancers and foulness of mouth"
5. *An Ethereal Amber*, "cures old rheumatism, spasms, cramps, palsies, old gouty callous swellings"
6. *Nervous Aethereal Balsam*, "the balmy bracer of weak nerves and relaxed fibres"
7. *Pectoral Balsam*, "for coughs, colds, asthmas, consumptions"
8. *The Solvent and Expeller*, for the "Gravel and Stone"
9. *British Drops*, a "safe, speedy, radical and infallible specific antidote against venereal disease in all its stages and degrees"
10. *The Bracing Balsam*, for the "effectual cure of gleets, feminal weakness, debility and impotency in men"
11. *Cephalic Powder*, a "safe, speedy and in general certain cure for fits"
12. *Aethereal Ambrosial Quintessence of Gold, Honey and Rosa Salis* for "nourishing and rejuvenating the body".[52]

As will be noted there is a certain overlap within the alleged therapeutic action of several of these medicines, but it would seem that the Nervous Aethereal Balsam and the Aethereal Ambrosial Quintessence were undoubtedly marketed as rejuvenants. The latter was obviously Dr. Graham's (he gave himself a gratuitous M.D., like many of his fellow quacks) favourite. "The discovery, right preparation and perfecting of this most noble, most truly divine medicine" was Graham's chief concern, readers are told in one of the handbills.

> For upwards of ten years . . . it was chiefly with a view of bringing this favourite project to the highest excellency of perfection and

usefulness that I hesitated not to expend upwards of twelve thousand pounds sterling in constructing and embellishing an Adepti-Alchyirical Medico-electrical and Philosophic Apparatus, infinitely superior to anything that now is or that ever was in the World.[52]

In a later pamphlet it is obvious that Graham had decided for the time being to concentrate all his energies on rejuvenation, for he now described only three medicines "prepared and dispensed" at the Temple of Health: Electrical Aether, Nervous Aethereal Balsam and Imperial Pills, all of which were marketed as potent rejuvenants.

The former were prepared:

> . . . in the great metal globes on the dome of the Electrical Temples of Health and of Hymen in the Apollo and other apartments . . . to be acted upon by the celestial fire. The essence is purified by filtration upon a new principle, which prevents all possibility of the finest and most volatile parts evaporating. The globes are entirely lined with metal on the in- as well as the outside. They are twelve in number, each containing full thirty-six gallons. The glass vessels too are covered with metal, enclosed in curious magnetic cases, and their stoppers are pierced with glass tubes and thick metal rods, which end in a multitude of points, from which streams of the electrical fire etc., are continually pouring in upon the aether and aromatics, in luminous and most glorious streams.[53]

Graham's ordinary medicines, sold stoppered up in the "best flint bottles" were never cheap, being marketed at five shillings and fivepence, two shillings and eightpence and "fifteen pence" a vial. The quintessences and rejuvenation medicines were considerably more expensive at a guinea a vial. On top of this, visitors at the Temple had to pay an admission fee that, according to contemporary newspapers, varied from one shilling to five shillings.[54] For this they were privileged to hear Graham's views on rejuvenation, and a fair amount of good sound sense on the general subject of hygiene.

From the point of view of Public Health, Graham was far in advance of his times. In an age when personal cleanliness was so rare that women often wore "ladies' flea traps", full of honey, under their voluminous skirts, Graham advocated the frequent airing of clothes and bedclothes. "All your wearing apparel too, as well as your bedclothes, should be hung on lines to blow about day and night in the wind and sun". He also advocated "washing the face, neck, hands, arms, feet, legs, private parts and fundament with pure, cold rain, river or soft open spring water", night and morning. He advised a simple mixed diet, the wearing of light-weight clothing, regular exercise, and the custom of husband and wife sleeping apart on occasions.

"Do not sleep every night with your wife or your husband . . . but let there be two beds in the room, or rather sleep in adjacent apartments, and at all times be seldom and moderate in your conjugal sacrifices", Graham frequently told his audiences.

At a somewhat later date, and probably during the year of 1781, Graham started to advertise yet another attraction at the Temple of Health. This was the "Grand Celestial or Magnetic-electrico Bed", made for Graham by the celebrated tinsmith, Denton. Housed in a special room, with convenient discrete access from the street, it was a rejuvenation apparatus, according to Graham, of unexcelled excellence.

The Grand Celestial Bed, whose magical influences are now cele-brated from pole to pole and from the rising to the setting of the sun, is 12ft. long by 9ft. wide, supported by forty pillars of brilliant glass of the most exquisite workmanship, in richly variegated colours. The super-celestial dome of the bed, which contains the odoriferous, balmy and ethereal spices, odours and essences, which is the grand reservoir of those reviving invigorating influences which are exhaled by the breath of the music and by the exhilarating force of electrical fire, is covered on the other side with brilliant panes of looking glass.

On the utmost summit of the dome are placed two exquisite figures of Cupid and Psyche, with a figure of Hymen behind, with his torch flaming with electrical fire in one hand and with the other, supporting a celestial crown, sparkling over a pair of living turtle doves, on a little bed of roses.

The other elegant group of figures which sport on the top of the dome having each of them musical instruments in their hands, which by the most expensive mechanism, breathe forth sound correspond-ing to their instruments, flutes, guitars, violins, clarinets, trumpets, horns, oboes, kettledrums etc.

The post or pillars too, which support the grand dome are groups of musical instruments, golden pipes, etc., which in sweet concert breathe forth celestial sounds, lulling the visions of Elysian joys.

At the head of the bed appears sparkling with electrical fire a great first commandment: *Be Fruitful, Multiply and Replenish the Earth.* Under that is an elegant sweet-toned organ in front of which is a fine landscape of moving figures, priest and bride's procession entering the Temple of Hymen.

In the Celestial Bed no feather bed is employed, but sometimes mattresses filled with sweet new wheat or oat straw mingled with balm, rose leaves, lavender flowers and oriental spices. The sheets are of the richest and softest silk, stained of various colours suited to the complexion. Pale green, rose colour, sky blue, white and purple, and are sweetly perfumed in oriental manner with the tudor rose, or with rich gums or balsams.

The chief principle of my Celestial Bed is produced by artificial lodestones. About 15 cwt. of compound magnets are continually pouring forth in an everflowing circle.

The bed is constructed with a double frame, which moves on an axis or pivot and can be converted into an inclined plane.

Sometimes the mattresses are filled with the strongest, most springy hair, produced at vast expense from the tails of English stallions, which are elastic to the highest degree.[55]

The Celestial Bed was supported by six massive brass pillars and covered with "saxon blue and purple satin drapes and perfumed with Arabian spices in the style of those in the Seraglio of a Grand Turk". Music was provided for those who wished to partake of "superior ecstasy which the parties enjoy in the Celestial Bed". The fee required by Graham for a night spent in this extraordinary contraption was £50.

Eventually at some time towards the end of 1781 Graham moved his headquarters to a new Temple of Health at Shomberg House, Pall Mall, where he practised rejuvenation therapy with assiduity for a further two years. It may have been an advertising "gimmick" to address his advertisements and handbills at this time to "Their Excellencies, the Foreign Ambassadors, the Nobility, Gentry and persons of learning and taste", and to mention that "during the last evenings an overflow of at least 900 ladies and gentlemen", but there is good evidence by the amount of publicity spontaneously given to Graham in contemporary newspapers and magazines that he was a very popular rejuvenator.

Like many famous men, Graham was soon to experience the public's fickleness and eventually he found himself out of favour. Unhappily the day came when the Temple of Health had to be closed and its famous contents sold. Incredibly there are no records extant of what became of Graham's electrical machines or the famous and bizarre Celestial Bed. For a while Graham supported himself with a new rejuvenation method, invented by himself and christened earth bathing. Taking a small house in Panton Street, then a popular area for sweathouses and dubious public bathing establishments of all sorts, Graham had himself immersed in earth while he gave lectures on the benefits of his new discovery. According to the contemporary scandal sheet, *The Ramblers Magazine*, he also persuaded young ladies as well to "bathe" quite naked in earth for the edification of the passing trade.

Quite soon, however, it became obvious that James Graham, greatest of the eighteenth-century quack rejuvenators, was approaching mental derangement. Although he still performed in many places throughout the British Isles, until nearly the end of the century, his practice deteriorated as did his wits and his unique ideas on rejuvenation.

From the point of view of ethical ideas in rejuvenation the early nineteenth century had little new to offer that is worthwhile recording. Nevertheless advances in Chemistry and Medical Science acted to a certain extent upon the mind of the quack. By the end of the century and the beginning of the twentieth century a basic environment of great promise was available to potential unethical rejuvenators.

Broadly speaking, rejuvenation was now offered in two ways. Firstly, there was "new youth" and restored body function, generally as a result of nerve tonics and various elixirs of life. The popularity of these compounds was probably due to imperfect lay understanding of the various pharmaceutical and scientific discoveries of the day. Secondly, there were the confident offers of sexual rejuvenation.

Two examples of the general body rejuvenating substances were "Phosferine" and "Sanatogen". The former was analysed by the scientists of the British Medical Association as early as 1912, when it was described by its manufacturers as a "potent strengthening medicine". The contents turned out to be a solution of 8 per cent alcohol in water containing a little quinine and sulphuric acid, to which had been added a dilute solution of phosphoric acid. The ingredients were estimated to cost less than 2 per cent of its retail price. "Sanatogen" was initially advertised in the *London Graphic* as "The Life food and nerve tonic, Rejuvenates and Revitalises", and was publicly endorsed by named members of parliament, bishops, other revered gentlemen, together with a fair sprinkling of the current peerage. When analysed "Sanatogen" proved to be merely powdered casein. Its manufacturers claimed among other things that "Sanatogen contained over 700 per cent more tissue building, life sustaining nourishment than wheat flour", and this encouraged dieticians of the American Medical Association to analyse a host of food materials and to compare them with "Sanatogen". Their findings were expressed crudely but effectively in a statement that "one dollar's worth of wheatflour contains as much energy as one hundred and ninety-seven dollars worth of 'Sanatogen' ". Of course, just because it was proved that the manufacturers of these foods were making enormous profits from their products was neither here nor there. If it were possible to show that the ingredients of either "Sanatogen" or "Phosferine" were responsible for rejuvenation it mattered not a jot what the profit margin was. But no independent scientific evidence has ever been produced that proves these products rejuvenate in the strictly medical sense, although people may feel better after taking them. The present day manufacturers of these and some other remedies are of course absolved from any implications of quackery and advertise their products in a thoroughly responsible way. Nor would the implication apply to the many reputable products now on the market and claimed by their makers to improve the sense of well-being.

Another early twentieth-century product, marketed under the impressive title of "Vitae Ore" illustrated once again that most rejuvenation ideas have their roots in antiquity. This powder, said to have been discovered by a nebulous Professor Theo Noel, a "well known geologist", was passed off as "a deposit from a marvellous medicinal spring". Advertised as being able to turn worn-out people into those with "vigour to spare, men with breezy personalities and women whose warm blood and feminine grace captures all hearts", it was found on analysis to consist of two very prosaic inorganic compounds, ferric oxy-sulphate and Epsom salt. Hardly more exciting pharmacologically were products like "Cocaphos", "puts new life in you, Invigorates, creates blood, nerve force and energy", "Neurovril", "Has the Elixir of Life been discovered? . . . old men and women made young, the yellow hued cheeks assume the roses of youth", of "Osoge", "containing the amazing elemental combination Seru-Phos".

Perhaps the most amusing food rejuvenant was "Antineuras-thin", an invention of a German physician, Dr. Hartmann, and introduced into Britain just prior to the 1914–18 war. Antineuras-thin was marketed and advertised as a cure for the "twentieth-century Disease", defined as a complicated syndrome that began with extensive sensitivity and might end in suicide. Dr. Hart-mann's discovery prevented and cured this disease and built up the "perfect balance of mental and physical power which alone can uphold health and happiness". Its proprietors believed it to be of "great interest to brain workers in all walks of life". When the British Medical Association decided to analyse this great continental therapeutic boon [56] they found it consisted of dried egg powder compressed into tablet form with a little dried potato water and lactose. From the point of view of nutritional value each tablet was equivalent to a teaspoon of fresh egg.

But if selling dried egg at an enormous profit was a German idea of great audacity, it pales before the technique of G. H. Brinkler, the self-designated "food expert" from Washington, D.C. In a nutshell Brinkler's thesis was that almost all disease processes, including ageing, are due to incorrect dietary habits. He, and only he, really understood these secrets of nature. But being a generous person he was willing to spread his unique know-ledge, at a price (usually seventy-five dollars), and so rejuvenation was within the reach of all.

Brinkler obtained the services of an Englishman, William H. Morse, M.D., to write his most impressive testimonials and advised potential patients that they "should remember his address in the hour of approaching death" for in all probability he could help at even this late time. Brinkler was, of course, an ill-educated quack of the worst possible type (one of his foibles was an expressed belief that butter caused deafness), but nevertheless he is worth remembering as a pioneer in the "food will do it" school of rejuvenation quackery.

Brinkler made a modest fortune before the US Post Office Department issued a fraud order against him. The proprietors of another American rejuvenation potion, "Sargol", pilfered from the American public some three million dollars before they too were prosecuted and fined 30,000 dollars.[57] "Sargol", marketed at first as a body-builder, soon became advertised as a rejuvenator for "thin, run-down men and women". It actually contained therapeutically worthless hypophosphites and a small dose of strychnine in the form of nux vomica. Essentially similar, as far as their pharmacological identity was concerned, were the once famous "Glow of Life" tablets, marketed by the Life Laboratories Company of Columbus, Ohio. Once again the American Postmaster General, utterly convinced that the "Fountain of Youth" did not really flow in the city of Columbus, issued a fraud order and another quack rejuvenation racket was smashed.

One idea that is fairly certain to succeed in any quack rejuvenation scheme is to claim that the secret remedy your particular nostrum contains, comes from far away places. In the same way as Dr. Hartmann's antineurasthin gained popularity because of its German origin, an American compound with the exotic name "El Zair" was advertised as containing ingredients "that could only be procured in certain lofty and almost inaccessible mountain ranges in Africa". To gild the lily is an everyday decorative process in quackery and the manufacturers, who hailed from prosaic West 16th Street, New York City, claimed that El Zair had, to boot, been elaborated by "an English scientist of considerable note", who in turn had been put on the trail of the rejuvenant from an Arabic manuscript that "came into the hands of a friend".

Provided the active principle of El Zair was harvested correctly "under certain phases of the moon" and compounded with certain mystical rites, the manufacturers claimed it to be a powerful pharmacological substance. It grew hair on bald heads, made barren women fertile, cured consumption, as well as "clearing away the deeper seated waste matter" that was the cause of old age. American Medical Association scientists, however, an incredulous body of men in the 1920s, found they could make a substance identical to "El Zair" in every way without going to Africa or, for that matter, leaving their laboratories in North Dearborn Street, Chicago, by merely dissolving two and half ounces of Epsom salt in a pint of distilled vinegar.

Sometimes the activities of the quacks who operated so successfully in this field combined two or more of the basic ideas of rejuvenation. For instance, the promoter of a botanical remedy called "Orchis Extract", by the name of Fred A. Leach of Chicago, started his business by selling purely mechanical "vacuum developers for the enlargement of the male organ". But, by and large, quacks kept to their own speciality pretty tightly. An example *par excellence* of mechanical aids to sexual rejuvenation was made by the Sanden Electric Company of Broadway, New York City, which sold an "electric belt" guaranteed to "restore Manhood". Electricity could, the manufacturers explained, do more than drugs in the matter of rejuvenation. Advertisements showed the virile man, a possessor of the famous belt, capturing the most attractive women at social occasions and leading a life that was a long and delicious amble along the road of eternal youth.

To all accounts the Sanden Electricity Company did well enough before they were eventually stopped using the US mails. Their overhead expenses in the manufacture of cheap and ordinary belts plus their sales organization cannot have been heavy. But one American rejuvenation quack thought out a method of getting around even these normal calls on a manufacturer's pocket by the simple expedient of selling advice. Briefly this was how to "recover and retain your youthful vigour and vitality without dangerous drugs or appliances". For a mere dollar the "copyrighted method" was dispatched to the client. This was said to work through "increasing the blood and nerve supply of the testicles ... by placing one hand on each side of the scrotum above the testicles and stretching them (the testicles) away from the body, moving the hands from side to side in a swaying motion while pulling". Surprisingly this confidence trick won many advocates before it was banned from using the US mails.[58]

Another practitioner of physical advice in the field of rejuvenation was Alois P. Swoboda of New York City, who was an early practitioner of the type of exercise rejuvenation later exploited to the full by Charles Atlas and others. Swoboda operated under a "ninety-day guarantee", to "restore youth to you, regardless of how old you are". "I guarantee to eradicate old age completely and permanently" the proprietor asserted. The course was immediately popular even in view of the twenty dollar fee.

The Swoboda system was simplicity itself. Removed from the devious phraseology so often found in quack literature, it involved flexing and relaxing certain muscles, a process recently graced with the descriptive title of isometrics. Somehow this, the rejuvenator felt, produced the "scientific antagonization of the energies and forces residing in the positive and negative cells of the brain, nervous system and muscles. . . . The antagonism of muscles is, in reality, more than 95 per cent of the potential element of my system". The simple physiological principle that it is virtually impossible to flex one's muscular system without relaxing its antagonizers seemed to have been completely overlooked by Swoboda's patients and despite the obvious "purity of his systematology" the "system" was a vastly profitable idea both for its orginator and his subsequent imitators.

It is impossible to leave the subject of physical rejuvenation ideas without a brief reference to Hercules Sanche who modestly described himself as the "Discoverer of the Laws of Spontaneous Cure of Disease", before he moved into his real *forte*, which was rejuvenation. Sanche's therapy for all disease consisted of strapping to ankle, leg, wrist or any other convenient part of the anatomy a flat piece of metal from which various pieces of wire sprouted. These, in turn, were connected to what for all intents and purposes was a piece of regulation metal gas pipe, usually filled with charcoal. Sanche's original "instrument", the Electro-poise, was modestly claimed to provide an "oxygen home remedy without medicine", that "supplies the needed amount of electric force to the system, and by its thermal action places the body in condition to absorb oxygen through the lungs and pores". Heartened by the success of this extraordinary piece of apparatus Sanche evolved the Oxydonor. This cost thirty-five dollars and was, therefore, three and a half times as expensive as the Electro-poise. Nevertheless its action was alleged to be far more potent. As well as "forcing" the body to absorb more oxygen it harnessed a new power—Diaductive Force.

The Force of Diaduction, another of Sanche's "inventions", was never explained. The inventor himself tried to explain it in a 468-word sentence, but somehow he did not succeed. Eventually when he was prosecuted Mr. Justice Shiras, a Supreme Court Judge, said, "I am entirely certain that I do not understand the working of this so-called Force, if any exists, and I greatly doubt whether Dr. Sanche has any clear conceptions of the Force or principle which he seeks to describe under the name of Diaduc-tion".

Whether or not the Force ever was explained or understood remains in doubt. Sanche was quite clear that it "revitalizes human beings, or animals or plants, to any required degree, as quickly as if accomplished by magic, while the patient feels little or nothing, and sleeps sweetly and naturally to wake in health, strong, vigor-ous, hungry and more highly animated than usual".[59] Sanche eventually developed the Force of Diaduction into a kind of religion, his converts swearing the Vow of Duxanimae, and inci-dentally making considerable contributions to Sanche's personal expenses in running his rejuvenation business. These, the inventor or high priest made quite sure had to be in the form of "conver-tible donations" to the "fund of the Cause of Duxanimae by Induction".

Naturally the Oxydonor had many subsequent imitators, the Oxytonor, the Oxypathor and the Oxyton, to mention only a few. Even in the 1930s a curiously reminiscent piece of apparatus on sale was the "Vitalizer" which comprised a simple flashlight, from which a cord was attached to a piece of metal the size of a pencil. This "element" was inserted into the rectum, the current switched on and electric force was supposed to flood the whole body.

Apart from, but often concomitant with general rejuvenation techniques ran sexual rejuvenation pure and simple. So deep is the desire in modern society to remain sexually potent to an advanced age that the fortune of any nostrum manufacturer is virtually secure if he hits upon and exploits a suitable sexual rejuvenation idea.

One of the most popular rejuvenation remedies in Britain for over fifty years has been a compound sold under the name of "Damaroids". Their original claim was that they marketed "a safe and sure cure for general weakness, physical decay, and loss of nerve power, varicocele etc.". Pharmacologically "Damaroids" are very simple. They contain hypophosphites of iron and quinine, substances of no specific rejuvenating or aphrodisiac nature. Their name seems to have been taken from a minute trace of extract of damiana that they contain.

More obvious in its claims, but nowhere near as successful over the years was "Gordon's Sexual Restorative",—a "viro-erectile Elixir" that was equally inert pharmacologically. Many other similar therapeutic confidence tricks existed, so similar to one another that little can be learnt of the basic ideas of rejuvenation by their study.

An exception to this statement must be made with reference to one classic idea in the history of sexual rejuvenation. It can best be explained in a phrase that, once coined, was used over and over again with great commercial success for well over a hundred years—"Lost Manhood". Exactly who can claim the doubtful honour of inventing this phrase is problematical. The idea behind "Lost Manhood", however, originated in the work of an English quack of the 1790 era, Dr. William Brodum.

Brodum, like many quacks of the day, obtained his degree by purchase at the Marischal College of Aberdeen, for a fee of five guineas. Practising in the Blackfriars area of London, Brodum sold two nostrums, "The Nervous Cordial" and "Botanical

Syrup". Neither of these would imply rejuvenation, and were it not for a book written by Brodum in 1795,[60] the essence of his quackery would easily be missed.

In a nutshell Brodum's credo, as expressed, was this. As a result of masturbation, practised in youthful years, the individual becomes prematurely aged, weak and feeble. Unless something is done about this, very quickly, physical deterioration can be expected, and eventually the mind will follow the depressing fate of the body. Brodum's book, expecially volume two, is a nauseating account of the end products of lost manhood and lost womanhood that even in these days of licence in literature would probably fall foul of the Director of Public Prosecution's Office.

One bright light, naturally enough, runs through all Brodum's terrible case histories. Once the patient starts taking the Nervous Cordial or Botanical Essence, it hardly seems to matter which, rejuvenation, mental, physical and sexual soon follow. Considering the period, Brodum made a thorough success of his quackery. Large bottles of his medicine retailed at £5, and at the height of his fame there were eight agencies selling the nostrums in London and a further sixty scattered throughout Britain.

The idea that Brodum started, that of treating Lost Manhood, was eventually fully exploited in the US. The venue of such activity was mainly in establishments known as Medical Institutes. A few Medical Institutes existed in London at the end of the nineteenth century but their influence was not as powerful as their American counterparts. Broadly speaking, the Institutes were the lair of the quack, or the disreputable doctor with a dubious degree or diploma. In the US during the first two decades of the twentieth century most large cities housed somewhere in their midst, a Medical Institute. Sometimes these establishments used as a "front" a spurious medical museum, in which waxwork models demonstrated to clients the horrors of "Lost Manhood", and venereal disease. In other situations the Institute operated from a respectable-looking office and employed doctors of an inferior ilk, who were instructed to diagnose these disreputable diseases, and treat them, whether they existed in their patients or not.

The most energetic operators of the Medical Institutes were

undoubtedly Dr. Edward N. Flint, and the Drs. Reinhart who originally hailed from Chicago. They employed and controlled a vast ring of Institutes managed and staffed by doctors whose qualifications were often as dubious as their own. Luckily, contemporary newspaper reports have preserved first-hand verbatim reports from former managers of these Institutes that give some evidence of the techniques involved. One such former manager confided the following to a newspaperman:

> One day the buzzer sounded upstairs and we waited a long time for the patient to appear. When he didn't show up, I looked down the stairs and there was Compton almost carrying an old man up the stairs. We got him in the operating room. He had neither hair nor teeth, he was deaf and his sight was failing. Compton had talked him into the belief that the only reason he wasn't as young as he used to be was because he had lost his manhood and we were the only people who could restore it. He signed a contract for a course of treatments by which he thought we could rejuvenate him. Of course we had got the big initial fee, which insured his return for more treatments. We had to carry him down the stairs on the way out, but he went home with the belief for all his eighty-four years that he would be a boy again in a week.[61]

The same manager also told of the actual methods of rejuvenation. There were two "medicines" involved, one was simply coloured water ("Aqua Michiganus" was the doctor's usual prescription), or for those who needed stronger medicine, elixir simplex. The preparation of the latter was extremely simple. Four pounds of sugar were dissolved in two and two-fifths pints of pure alcohol and enough water added to make the fluid contents up to two gallons. Burnt sugar and orange essence coloured and flavoured the "medicine", which was sold for two to five dollars for a four-ounce bottle. As the "floor man" candidly remarked to *The Chicago Tribune*, "It is almost whisky and any man who uses it regularly can get a jag on it".

For those who presumably did not like medicine or did not respond to either of the Institute's stock mixtures, "Hinckle's Pills", a mild cathartic, were usually prescribed. ("We had them there in three colours, so that a patient could be kept using them three weeks".)

One of the associates of the Flint-Reinhart organization in Chicago was a Dr. B. M. Ross, who, incidentally, claimed to be "a regular physician who had twenty-five years of continuous practice in Chicago". He used to advertise regularly in three foreign languages in the newspapers, making sure that citizens who could not read English were catered for effectively. Other quacks specializing in cures for "self-wrecked men" used bogus electrical machines as part of their treatment.

One of the clever commercial ideas by means of which the unsuspecting were duped in the Medical Institutes has also been part and parcel of rejuvenation quackery in more modern times. This is the "free consultation" initially offered to patients. "I make no charge for counsel! Call!" middle-aged men were told by the proprietor of Wisconsin Medical Institute. "The springtime of youth has passed" and "looking back over your life you can point out the mistakes you have made . . . and nature will make no compromise in your case . . . the penalty is sickness, death and decay", a handbill told potential patients. But all was not lost. "Go to the Wisconsin Medical Institute and ask for help", the middle-aged were told . . . "Our wonderful electro medical treatment is saving thousands and will save you."[62]

Gradually, as a result of the activity of a more enlightened press, the activities of the American Medical Association and a slowly improving public knowledge of medical matters, the Medical Institutes fell out of favour and their patients dwindled, thus ending a fascinating though extremely disreputable era in the history of quack rejuvenation.

One of the most important rules of successful quackery is always to move with the times scientifically. In the 1930s there was widespread, if erroneous, public knowledge of the essentials of sexual rejuvenation by means of sex gland extracts and implants. It could hardly be expected that the quacks would overlook the opportunity to be explored in this profitable field of activity, and the man whose name was most closely linked with this activity was "Dr." John R. Brinkley.

Brinkley went to considerable trouble to establish himself as a "medical" man, without, of course, going through the necessary course of training. His premedical education, he claimed, was taken at Milton Academy, Baltimore, from whence he received his B.A. Unfortunately Milton Academy was a notorious Diploma Mill, whose "Dean" could claim fame through a six-month sentence in jail for fraud.[43] Then Brinkley obtained a LL.D. in another similar establishment, the Oskaloos College, Iowa. Feeling, perhaps, that there was a hiatus in his medical education, the future rejuvenator worked for a while at the Eclectic Medical University of Kansas City before graduating at another Diploma Mill, the Kansas City College of Medicine and Surgery. Eventually he became extremely powerful socially in Milford in the 1920s, and obtained a real licence to practise medicine in the State of Kansas.

A temporary setback in the career of this extraordinary medical man was an episode in 1920 when he was arrested for selling intoxicating liquors and maintaining a public nuisance in violation of the liquor laws of Kansas. Fined three hundred dollars and confined to jail for ninety days, Dr. Brinkley managed to persuade a judge to grant him a parole on payment only of the cost of the action against him.[63]

By now Brinkley's medical credo was fully established, and available from various medical institutions, for example, Brinkley Research Laboratories and the Brinkley-Jones Hospital Association incorporating the College of Physicians and Surgeons. There he practised transplantation of goat glands into ageing males,—his so-called "compound operation" and the injection rectally of his "special gland Emulsion". Brinkley, who boasted US Senators and other prominent people as his patients, lived up to the idea that to quack well you must quack expensively. The special gland injection cost a hundred dollars, while the operation cost from 750 to 1200 dollars, dependent upon the age of the goat!

Brinkley eventually made a bad mistake in applying to practise in California on the grounds of the reciprocity for his degrees, for by now he was claiming to be an M.D. and SC.D.! He had, apparently, already been operating in California for some time, having, he claimed, rejuvenated the managing editor of a Los Angeles newspaper. Unfortunately for him, the Californian authorities were completely unimpressed with his degrees, and diplomas, and refused to license him in their State, and were even unkind enough to apply for his extradition for conspiring to violate the medical laws of the State.

Luckily Brinkley's reputation and power in Kansas saved him, for the State Governor refused to honour the requisition. Gradually Brinkley's reputation tarnished even in Kansas. For many years he had owned his own radio station, from whence had originated all his quack claims to rejuvenation. Eventually, however, he lost his licence to broadcast. This did not worry him unduly, for he merely bought a station in Mexico and commuted in his private aircraft between Del Rio and Little Rock, Arkansas.

Brinkley's medical aspirations received a further setback when an Italian University that had for some reason given him an honorary degree revoked his qualification. But, by now the wealthy owner of four cars, several yachts and a private plane, he had outgrown the simple life of a rejuvenatior and decided to enter political life in earnest. On three occasions he ran for Governor of Kansas and on one occasion was only narrowly defeated. Before his death in 1937 Brinkley founded a hospital at Little Rock and a church in Milford. On the latter is the touching inscription, that tells visitors that it was "Erected to God and His Son Jesus in appreciation of the many blessings conferred upon me. J. R. Brinkley".[64]

Although Brinkley's ideas and methods have probably not been bettered as far as moden quackery is concerned, other keen but less successful operators also exploit glandular theories in rejuvenation, for instance the Medical Aid Bureau that sold "Golden Glan". This came in two forms, one for the male who "doesn't realize that he is not paying his wife the attention he formerly did" and another for women "to mould soft curves, give her ripe, red lips, rosy cheeks, and the fascinating claims of the feminine sex".

Similarly, the New Life Corporation sold gland capsules to "permanently cure impotency and waning sexual power". On analysis these were found to contain some glandular extract but also cantharides. Similarly, the Peptoro Medical Company advertised they could cure ninety-five out of one hundred cases of "Lost Manhood" by means of their gland extract, made up in combination with "a salt of pure gold and yohimbine". In actual fact the glandular preparations marketed by this company, organized not by a bogus doctor but by a retired lumberjack, contained cantharides, nux vomica and iron and ammonium citrate. Glands or their extracts, gold and yohimbine were conspicuous only on the label.

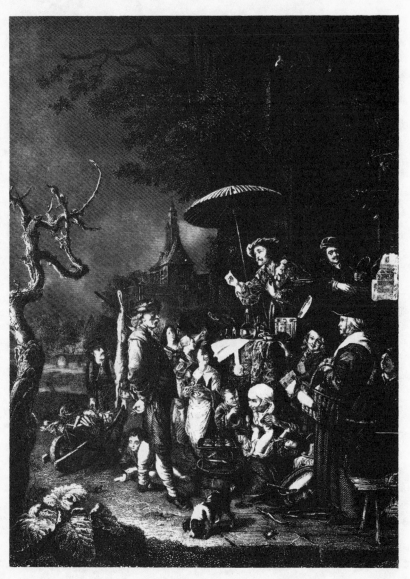

"The Quack Doctor"

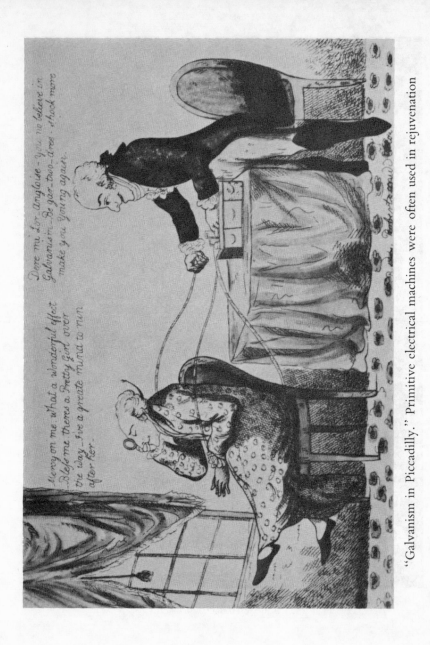

"Galvanism in Piccadilly." Primitive electrical machines were often used in rejuvenation

6

Metchnikoff and Intestinal Intoxication

Perhaps the first theory of rejuvenation ever to take the fancy of the world of science is one that will always be linked with the Russian biologist and Nobel prize-winner, Elie Metchnikoff. The rise and fall of the basic principles that lay behind Metchnikoff's theories, and the way they influenced other prominent contemporaries and eminent professional men who followed in the wake of his impetus must be examined with reference to both the personality of Metchnikoff and the scientific climatology at the turn of the century. Only then will it be possible to understand the genesis of the intoxication theory of ageing and the method of rejuvenation introduced, quite logically, to reverse such processes.

Metchnikoff was born on 16th May, 1845, and grew up in the Steppe region of Kharkoff, known as Little Russia, within an environment that might be described as near to the bottom rung of the aristocratic ladder. His father was an army officer, whose early days were spent in what had become accepted as the conventional behaviour of a young, married guardsman in the Imperial Army. When he had effectively gambled away his young wife's fortune at the tables at St. Petersburg, and had reduced the family fortunes to such an extent that a purely rural life was the only possible solution open to them, the basic die was cast that was to produce the future scientist and rejuvenationist.

Elie, the youngest of the family, grew up to become a fair and slender boy with a "diaphanous, pink and white complexion . . . small grey eyes, full of kindliness and sparkle. Very highly strung and impressionable, his temper easily roused, [who] always wished to see everything, know everything, and find his way every-where".[65]

Biographers telling of his early life draw attention to highly significant facts that are worth examining if we are to understand his later years. First of all he was very much a spoilt child and patently his mother's favourite. He suffered from a chronic ble-pharitis as a youngster and this was interpreted as "weakness" of the eyes by the family medical adviser who advocated, rather dogmatically perhaps, that young Elie must be saved tears at any price, as crying or tantrums always brought on an attack of "eye suffering".

The special position secured by the growing boy in his family as a result of this medical disability can easily be appreciated. His sister thought he was a "little beast" and one gathers that his elder brothers were not over-impressed with Elie as a country house companion. As a result he was very much the pet of the female servants, as well as his mother, to whom as a young man he was psychologically attached in a most abnormal and unhealthy way. In all probability these medical, domestic and environmental fac-tors combined in Metchnikoff to produce character defects liable to make a scientist's career rather unhappy. His personality combined obsessive tendencies, that at times assumed almost para-noid proportions, and emotional immaturity associated with depression.

At the age of eight fate provided an opportunity for the rather neurotic little boy, by now well fastened to his mother's apron-strings, to occupy his active young brain in some useful activity. His second eldest brother, Leo, had to be removed from school at St. Petersburg due to a hip complaint, an event which necessitated the engagement of a tutor for home study. Although Leo was an intelligent enough pupil, the tutor was more impressed with young Elie who, though so young, showed unusual intelligence in the study of natural science. Later when he was admitted to the Kharkoff Lycée, Elie started to consolidate his early scientific aspirations. Turning away from his family's religion to embrace the principles of atheism while still a student, he managed to strike up a relationship with the university lecturer in physiology, and finally passed from student years as a Gold Medallist.

Metchnikoff's early scientific life seems to have been a series of quite brilliant episodes, strongly interspersed, however, with periods of strange, neurotic and very inexplicable behaviour. For instance, he early established a new order of fresh water creatures, the Gastrotricha, evolutionarily halfway between the Rotifera and the Nematode Worms. He also made valuable contributions to comparative embryology. But one day on an impulse he decided to leave his studies at Kharkoff to go to Germany and the University of Wurtzburg. Unfortunately he arrived there in the middle of the vacation, and behaved in a curiously immature way, flying back to Kharkoff in dismay and alarm at his unfortunate experience. Another curious episode in his early career was when he took an assistantship under an eminent professor at Gottingen, with a view to studying vertebrate anatomy, but before he had been in the laboratory twenty-four hours surprised everyone by throwing a valuable dissection across the room in a fit of pique.

Already, too, there was evidence of strange periods of indisposition that seemed to be part and parcel of the future rejuvenator's way of life. Violent fits of giddiness often made him incapable of work. He easily became depressed. The previous "eye weakness" troubled him from time to time as well. Letters written to his mother at the time demonstrate the unnatural emotional tie between the two. Even the most superficial psychiatric assessment of Metchnikoff's relationship with the opposite sex suggests the conclusion that he was incapable of conventional normal male-female liaisons. His interest vacillated between women who approximated to his mother's age and very young girls years his junior. His first marriage was to one of the former, his second to a mere child. Fortunately his innate kindness to this young woman allowed her to learn to love him in a satisfactory way, and eventually she helped him with his scientific work and, at last, wrote his biography. Neither of his wives ever became pregnant.

It would seem probable that Metchnikoff's poor sexual adjust-ment was part of his neurotic personality. As he proceeded to live his important life as a naturalist and biologist, whenever an emo-tional upheaval or a particularly difficult situation arose the bearded Russian would retreat into his neurotic shell. He attemp-ted suicide on more than one occasion. At times he would lock himself up in a darkened room to "spare his eyes". After one such bout of depression he prescribed himself a special diet—hitting suddenly upon the idea that his current illness was the result of chronic poisoning by microbes in his intestine. It was at this moment that one of the most remarkable of all rejuvenation ideas, based on a scientific background, was conceived.

But to understand the eminent biologist's strange convictions we must examine Metchnikoff's career a little more carefully. His early work need not bother us too much, except for the fact that during his travels as a young man he had developed a strong liking for marine biology. The year 1881 was significant for the scientist, his wife and the history of rejuvenation. A short while previously he had tried to kill himself in a curious way by inoculating himself with relapsing fever. Not long after his mental and physical re-covery his wife's father died, leaving them a small estate. Life was not very happy in Little Russia at this time as a result of friction between the Government and the farmers and peasants. So the young couple (he was only thirty-six and looked "like a figure of Christ"), travelled to the shores of the Mediterranean. Soon Metchnikoff was again involved with his beloved marine biologi-cal studies.

It is often difficult to appreciate the train of thought that starts a scientist working on any specific theory. But Metchnikoff's initial idea, which helped to solve one of the most important pathological mysteries of our age, has been preserved in his own words. He had been making observations on the mobile meso-dermic cells of starfish.

One day . . . I remained alone with my microscope, observing the life of the mobile cells of a transparent starfish larva, when a new thought suddenly flashed across my brain. It struck me that similar cells might serve in the defence of the organism against intruders.

... I said to myself, if my supposition is true, a splinter introduced into the body of a starfish larva, devoid of blood vessels or of a nervous system, should soon be surrounded by mobile cells. ...

Metchnikoff proceeded to carry out the experiment, and early next day his preparation demonstrated the exact phenomenon postulated. It was only a short step intellectually to liken the behaviour of mesodermic leucocytes in higher animals during bacterial inflammation, to the mobile cells he had seen at work in the starfish. In 1883 he published his initial findings,[66] and a new chapter in the history of pathology had started.

Strangely, Metchnikoff did not originate the term "phagocyte" himself. The conception of an army of devouring cells throwing themselves at an invader was "invented" by some scientist friend of his, at his own instigation, and is merely a Greek translation of "devouring cells".

By means of a neat experiment the theory of the phagocytosis was shown to be strictly applicable to changes occurring in spontaneous diseases. This was carried out on the transparent fresh water crustacean, Daphnia, and demonstrated the way they reacted to infection with a parasitic fungus, Monospora Bicuspidata.[67] As might be expected such a revolutionary conception of the aetiology of disease processes did not receive universal appreciation. Several foremost scientific men of the day—including the great Robert Koch—opposed it bitterly. Gradually, however, Metchnikoff's disciples multiplied. Settling in Paris in 1888 he found Pasteur and his colleagues to be powerful allies. Soon Lister agreed with his theories and eventually the world bowed to his unique and proven ideas on the defence mechanisms against bacterial diseases.

Metchnikoff's struggle to gain worldwide recognition of his theory seems to have influenced his personality in two important ways. Firstly he believed even more firmly now that to understand any scientific process it is necessary to study the reactions of primitive organisms for essential clues that may point to further progress. Then comparative anatomy can be applied in furthering analogies to higher organisms. Secondly Metchnikoff's struggle against the opinions of his scientific peers developed his inherent excessive and abnormal sensibility to criticism into a state of mental behaviour that permitted him to follow any of his chosen ideas with obsessional dogmatism.

Shortly after a particularly stimulating and personally successful meeting of the International Congress that took place in Moscow in 1897, Metchnikoff devoted his attention once again to the functions of the large, wandering macrophages that he now knew were present in all tissues in varying numbers. He observed them ingesting damaged red corpuscles, spermatozoa and damaged somatic cells of almost every type. Sometimes the cells he studied had been weakened by developmental processes, for instance the absorption of the metamorphosing tadpoles tail, and sometimes by toxins, disease, or even the process of old age.

Metchnikoff had already developed ideas that led him to believe that ageing was due to cell "weakness" or abnormality and these seemed to fit in well with those so recently and universally approved with reference to phagocytosis. In short, the presence of certain organisms in the bowel allowed toxins to be absorbed into the circulation which permeated the whole organism, damaging somatic cells as they did so, and the macrophages ingested the so damaged cells. As a result, cellular depreciation of essential tissues occurred. Senility was the final outcome of this sequence of events.

Metchnikoff next proceeded to put his theory to the test of comparative anatomy, and as a result came to conclusions that supported his hypothesis. Many primitive marine creatures, especially those without a separate digestive system, he observed to live almost indefinitely. For example, a species called *Actina mesembryanthemum* had a recorded existence of sixty-six years and retained its reproductive activity fully throughout its life. Many other polyps behave in a similar way and seemed to confirm the established principle that a poorly differentiated or absent alimentary canal scores positively as far as longevity is concerned. Metchnikoff was also intrigued to find that certain molluscs, especially the gastropods, live similarly infinite lives and they too are noted for the simplicity of their digestive arrangements.

The difference between the lifespan of predatory birds and the flying kinds also seemed to fit in well with the idea that gut complexity and therefore potential stagnation and intoxication by organisms was reflected in comparative longevity. Birds like the ostrich approximate very much to mammals in relationship to their bowel complexity. Indeed, Metchnikoff argued effectively that animals that are naturally both the hunter and the hunted have an evolutionary advantage if they enjoy the facility of storing waste intestinal products in complicated and relative stagnant bowels until such time as they can conveniently be voided.

> I have formed the theory that the large intestine has been increased in mammals to make it possible for these animals to run long distances without having to stand still to defaecate. . . . Mammals have to move actively to hunt their prey or escape their enemies. . . . According to such a view, the extreme development of the large intestine would supply a real want in the struggle for existence. . . . Although the capacity of the large intestine may preserve the mammal energies, it is attended with disadvantages that may shorten the actual duration of life.[68]

The flying birds and mammals, however, have evolved in such a way that lightness is all-important to their biological economy. This being so, they have simple bowels that retain food products for a minimal period. Even tiny birds, like canaries and larks, can live for over twenty years in captivity—an enormous lifespan relative to their size—and much larger birds, like the swan and goose, can live to be seventy or eighty. Facts like these encouraged Metchnikoff to pursue a bowel detoxication system as a method of promoting longevity and favouring rejuvenation.

If Metchnikoff was at home exploring the complex world of comparative anatomy, he was uncomfortable in the not-so-scientific maze of medical pathology. In an attempt to find examples of human disease processes that could be laid at the door of intestinal intoxication, he often made wild mistakes.

Quoting a Dr. du Pasquier,[69] he gave the following signs and symptoms of constipation in children. "The infant is leaden in hue, with sunken eyes, dilated pupils and pinched nostrils. The temperature may reach nearly 104° F., the pulse is rapid, feeble and often irregular. Restlessness, insomnia, sometimes convulsions occur. Stiffness of the neck and strabism show that the nervous system is being poisoned by toxins." Although the "toxicity" of such a child could hardly be in doubt, a disease process rather more definite than constipation would seem highly likely. Similarly, he gave an accurate description of a strange illness that occurred after childbirth. "The patient is seized with chill and headache. The breath is fetid and the tongue furred. The temperature taken in the axilla is 101° F. The abdomen is inflated and painful in the umbilical region."[70] This would now seem clearly to have been a case of puerperal pyrexia, and nothing to do with the constipation that usually occurs in all fevers.

Had Metchnikoff enjoyed a wider experience of medical pathology he would doubtless have heard of the work of Ignaz Semmelweis at the Vienna Lying-In Hospital and the subsequent slow, but steady progress of ideas that led, eventually, to a thorough understanding of the problems of post-puerperal infection and sepsis. But by now the obsessional nature of Metchnikoff was propelling his life's energies into concocting theories about rejuvenation that were often based upon his often rather narrow and obsessive observations.

Illness was never far from Metchnikoff's everyday personal experience and when only fifty-three he was convinced that he had ageing kidneys. Naturally enough he decided to test his own theories and adopted a diet aimed at "avoiding noxious microbes" being absorbed into his body. This involved drinking sour milk and avoiding all uncooked food. Metchnikoff persevered with his treatment and his health greatly improved.

Eventually these theories became widely publicized and resulted in widespread interest in the drinking of sour milk, and later yoghourt. A manufacturer in Paris approached the now eminent scientist with a view to producing the rejuvenating substances on a commercial footing. Metchnikoff, utterly convinced of the youth-giving qualities of the soured milk (he was now sixty-seven), agreed, and arranged for some young scientific friends of his to handle this side of the business. The factory eventually went into action and soured milk was marketed by a firm who sold their product, with permission, as the "sole provider of Professor Metchnikoff".

Although the legal adviser of the Pasteur Institute, where Metchnikoff was currently working, agreed in principle to using the "guarantee of the name of Metchnikoff", this commercial enterprise, although leading to no personal profit for its protagonists, produced violent criticism in the press. Doubtless, the rather exuberant nationalism of the French at this time, during which foreigners had invaded the country in large numbers, and held many of the best jobs and most lucrative positions, all at a time of social crisis, fanned the flames of criticism. Nevertheless, the fact that an eminent professor had become associated with the world of industry was unthinkable in the early days of the century.

But Metchnikoff was unabashed and passionately and obsessionally believed in his theory. When he was seventy he wrote of his "reduced orthobiosis", brought about by eating no raw food for eighteen years and having introduced as many lactic acid bacilli into his intestines as possible. He only regretted his limited success, complaining, "in spite of all, I am being poisoned by the bacteria of butyric fermentation". The great biologist died slowly and bravely in 1916, not as the result of any intoxication but due to congestive heart failure. There is little evidence that the theory of rejuvenation by bowel detoxication lost any ground as a result of his demise, for there were many powerful advocates to speak, act and write in support of his ideas.

Even before Metchnikoff's death there was much discussion in perfectly respectable medical circles on the pros and cons of intestinal intoxication. As early as 1913 the Royal Society of Medicine held a six-meeting symposium on the subject, in which no fewer than fifty speakers put their points of view. As far as can be judged from letters in contemporary medical journals, the profession in Britain was split on the true significance of the condition. Strangely perhaps, Metchnikoff's teachings appealed to surgeons rather than physicians and the former found they could make tremendous improvements in their patients' health and vitality by putting Metchnikoff's anatomical theories into practice. As a result, some thousands of patients had literally hundreds of yards of their large bowel removed on surgical advice.

It must not be assumed that such surgical feats were carried out by men of less than first-class professional standing. The most notable advocate was W. Arbuthnot Lane, F.R.C.S., Surgeon to Guy's Hospital and Senior Surgeon to Great Ormond Street Hospital. Lane referred to intestinal stasis as a chronic form of poisoning, and described its signs and symptoms, that in many cases were identical with those of premature ageing. They included "A progressive loss of fat and increased staining of the skin that made it inelastic, thin, plastic, abnormally dark and dirty looking". This was, Lane thought, especially noticeable in women in the "neck, eyelids and the cheeks, whose breasts also underwent degenerative changes". Lane's Disease, as the syndrome later became called, was also believed to predispose to cancer, tuberculosis, rheumatoid arthritis, gout and ulcers, as well as faintness, giddiness, neuralgia, headache and general lack of *joie de vivre*.

Sometimes, well known physicians allied themselves to the auto-intoxication theory of disease and premature ageing. One of the foremost was Sir James Mackenzie, the cardiologist, who clearly thought that his so-called "X" disease of the heart (now referred to as a D.A.H. or cardiac neurosis), was produced by intestinal auto-intoxication. Specialists in other fields of medical practice also felt they could see intestinal poisoning claiming their patients' health prematurely. Ernest Clark, F.R.C.S., a prominent ophthalmic surgeon of the early years of the century was convinced that intestinal toxaemia produced "hardening of the lens" with defective vision similar to that seen in old age. For a while there was immense enthusiasm for the Lane type of surgical rejuvenation.

But the 1930s saw the end of "short circuit operations" to rescue people from the terrors of intestinal stasis and auto-intoxication. By now the real reason for such operations had moved far from ideas of rejuvenation proper. Here and there, however, pockets of resistance, probably still influenced albeit unconsciously by Metchnikoff's theories, persisted. Sir Henry M. W. Gray of

Montreal was, in 1936, still very pleased with the results of his modified Lane operation that he called "abdominal spring cleaning". The great Sir Arbuthnot, however, had moved away from the active world of surgery to found the New Health Society and spread the gospel of positive health brought about by fresh air, adequate food, and significantly, proper and regular action of the bowels by means of prodigious quantities of liquid paraffin.

Today British surgeons have abandoned operations for intestinal stasis, fully in accordance with Sir Adolphe Abrahams' expression of opinion in the current *Encyclopedia of Surgical Practice* that such a condition never existed.

The books on the health-giving and rejuvenating effects of lactic acid bacteria, whether they be taken in cheese, sour milk or yoghourt, are largely unread today and the latter has become a pleasant dessert sold by the milk roundsmen, mainly for children to consume.

Metchnikoff would have been immensely stimulated by the modern pharmacological revolution. Probably the psychotrophic drugs now used with such great effect in a variety of psychological illnesses would have helped his psychopathic personality to adjust itself more adequately to its environment. Antibiotics have been developed—and particularly the broad spectrum ones taken by mouth—which are capable within a few hours of sterilizing the contents of the whole bowel. Nobody has ever felt any younger after this procedure which is often found to be a disadvantage for now we realize that the normal intestinal flora are essential to health and comfort. Significantly the taking of yoghourt together with broad spectrum antibiotics or shortly after them, obviates many of the symptoms of diarrhoea and intestinal discomfort that follow intensive antibiotic therapy, due, in all probability, to the vast number of lactic acid bacteria that it contains.

7

Cellular Therapy

Even in the hands of the most competent surgeon every operation has its own inherent hazards and complications. When it is necessary to remove the thyroid gland, either for simple or toxic goitre, there is always the possibility that parathyroid tissue may be excised accidentally together with the offending thyroid. There are several reasons for this. Sometimes the four tiny parathyroids glands that usually rest on the deep surface of the thyroid are abnormally placed. They may be adherent, or even embedded in thyroid tissue and the most careful surgical dissection may fail to reveal their position at operation.

This state of affairs possibly existed when, at Berne Clinic in 1931, an unknown surgeon carried out an over-enthusiastic thyroidectomy, and during the post-operative period his patient began to show first the irritability and apprehension, and later the abnormal sensations and muscular cramps that are recognized as the early signs of parathyroid tetany. Today, treatment with intravenous calcium and parathyroid hormone would soon control the condition, but in the early thirties such a complication was often the harbinger of a particularly painful death.

Faced with this previously mentioned crisis the Clinic called their director, Professor de Quervain. He confirmed the diagnosis and instituted remedial therapy, all without any substantial improvement in the patient, who continued to experience painful and increasingly severe tetanic cramps. It became obvious that the case would in all probability end fatally, but at this depressing juncture Professor de Quervain remembered the work of a young surgeon who lived nearby in Montreux and who had recently published papers on a particularly *avant garde* subject—the grafting of animal glands on to human tissues.[71] Feeling, perhaps, that desperate conditions warranted desperate remedies, the man in question, Paul Niehans, was contacted. He agreed to help.

After seeing the patient Niehans was not very hopeful. "As the patient arrived in a moribund condition, I could not even consider a surgical transplantation . . . so I cut the parathyroid of an ox into tiny pieces, made a suspension with physiological saline solution and injected it into the pectoral muscles of the patient."[72] Apparently Professor de Quervain was quite horrified at this procedure, expressing a fundamental criticism that all subsequent medical men have echoed, that is, that the injection of large quantities of "foreign" protein into the body would doubtless be followed by the severe sensitivity reaction of anaphylactic shock. But no such reaction occurred. Niehans had expected to make subsequent injections, or perhaps if his patient's condition improved, to carry out a classical implantation operation. But so dramatic was the sick man's response that soon it was obvious the crisis had passed.

Niehans subsequently related that he experienced a flash of understanding when the patient first showed signs of recovery. He deduced, perhaps erroneously, that the live parathyroid cells he had injected proliferated in the body and made up for the deficiency of internal secretion. In any case the year 1931 will be remembered for the birth of Niehan's Cellular Therapy— or, as he afterwards called it, the "implantation of organs by injection"—and a controversy had begun that even today has not been effectively settled.

Niehans stands as possibly the most famous of all professional rejuvenators. Quoting Goethe, "We live as long as God has ordained, but there is a great difference between living wretchedly, like poor dogs, and being well and vigorous", Niehans did his best to put the poet's ideas into practice. As a direct result he has surrounded himself with a unique entourage of patients.

Although there is no real evidence to support the rumour, and indeed Niehans makes no personal claims to the fact, it is widely believed that he was called into consultation with other eminent physicians and surgeons when the late King George VI of Great Britain was found to be suffering from enteritis.

It would seem reasonably certain, however, that Niehans treated the most elite, including one of India's most powerful princes, the Rajah of Darbhanga. His disease was described by Niehans as neuro-vegetative dystonia. Judging by the symptoms, this would appear to be a simple, endogenous depression associated with insomnia and impotence, rather than simply a "cocktail of ennui", a description given to the syndrome by Niehans' biographer.[73] Niehans injected placental and testicular cells and obtained a favourable response within his specified period of three weeks.

Later in his successful career Niehans rejuvenated many notable personalities, including Winston Churchill, Dr. Adenauer, Bernard Baruch the financier, Gloria Swanson and Furtwangler the famous conductor. Somerset Maugham gave the *News of the World* his permission to report his own recourse to Niehans in 1964, when the celebrated author was aged ninety. Not only did Maugham apparently benefit from the treatment but his secretary, Alan Searle, who also took the cure, felt so young afterwards that he was "ready to climb trees with anyone".

Niehans obviously felt his finest hour to be when he was called to see Pope Pius XII, an occurrence that supported him at a particularly difficult time, as will be apparent later.

When assessing the success that eminent medical men have with their patients, it is important to inquire into the nature of their personality as well as the method of treatment involved, for in all probability one is profoundly influenced by the other. A quick glance at Niehans' background makes it clear that he was born well-fitted both socially and temperamentally to be the physician and confidant of the very great.

His father, as a young surgeon of twenty-eight and already established in Berne, fell under the charm of a seventeen-year-old girl called Anna Kaufmann, who lived locally as the ward of a German family in the city. To his astonishment, on application to Miss Kaufmann's guardians he discovered that the blue blood of the Hohenzollerns ran very much in her veins, for Anna was no less than one of the several illegitimate children of the late King Frederick III, whose son Wilhelm II (in future to be known as the Kaiser), was already on the throne of Germany. It must be pointed out that although this story is told by all of Niehans' biographers, and confirmed by Niehans himself, it is quite absent from the standard historical reference books and contemporary records available in this country. Nevertheless Paul Niehans' subsequent behaviour seems to substantiate the story.

Kaiser Wilhelm appears to have been generously inclined towards his young half-sister, for he sent his ambassador to her wedding in Berne Cathedral, and blessed the union with a substantial income for life. (Incidentally, Anna Niehans is thought to have paid back her half-brother's friendliness and generosity by making several secret journeys for him within the safety of her Swiss nationality during the débâcle of 1917–18.)

The young couple had only one son, Paul. To all accounts he was a very bright boy. A letter written by a professor of mathematics is extant,[73] stating "Gifts of this quality are not often met with. We take the liberty of calling your attention to the importance of encouraging your son to advance as far as possible in the study of mathematics". Significantly the eulogy closed with the words, "The power of his imagination can rapidly lead him to the limits of human knowledge".

Young Niehans was not only a brilliant scholar, but an excellent shot, both with the gun and bow. He was also a first-class horseman. At the age of seventeen he was quite convinced that he should attend the Officer School in Potsdam to serve as a guard in a Regiment of Kaiser Wilhelm II. But the wise counsel of his parents prevailed and he eventually entered a seminary becoming a Doctor of Theology by the time he was twenty-one. Neihans at this time is described as a young, blond giant with steely blue eyes, winning the acclamation of Berne with his charm, intelligence and fervour.

The young pastor, however, found his life as a Doctor of Theology unsatisfactory. Influenced perhaps by his father, he decided to renounce the church for a career in medicine. Niehans as a medical student is described as a "wildly social playboy", gracing every elegant party that came his way and drinking at taverns until the dawn in the best spirit of the early twentieth century.

His early medical career is of little interest as far as his subsequent work as a rejuvenator is concerned, and his military career was punctuated with episodes that showed the extreme self-confidence of the man and his intolerance with those he considered his intellectual or social inferiors. On one occasion as a young Second Lieutenant he presented himself impudently and unasked before the Kaiser, who was said to be both surprised and delighted at the youthful officer's audacity, and insisted upon Niehans joining his staff as an *aide* for a short period. Eventually, after several years' experience as a medical officer and surgeon in the Army, that often proved embarrassing when various foreign authorities discovered his close relationship to the German monarch, Niehans ended his military career to enter private practice. Quite soon he was much in demand in a very specialized field of surgery, that of glandular implantation. Gradually he extended his activities and in 1931 the important glandular injection was carried out that provided the turning point in Niehans' extraordinary career.

There were many contributory factors in Niehans' decision to devote himself to the personally hazardous and extraordinary career of rejuvenator. His natural Hohenzollern arrogance and drive was but one of them. A fortunate inheritance of a considerable income on his mother's death was another. Perhaps the extremely varied experience in early life was a symptom of an almost obsessional dislike for routine. But in all events a purpose more thrilling than mundane surgical practice spurred Niehans on in the period that followed his "awakening" in 1931, and within a few years he was completely involved in cellular therapy.

Slowly he elaborated the method and the criteria that had

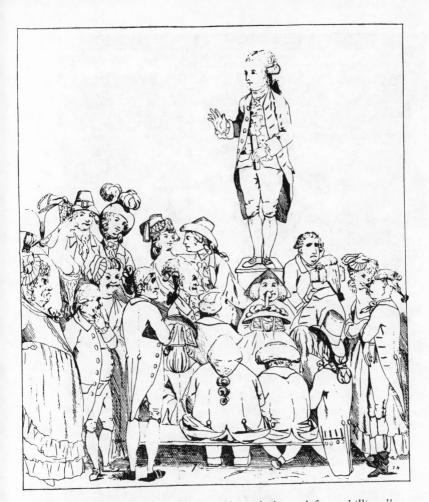

"The doctor himself pouring out his whole soul for a shilling."
One of the few pictures extant of Dr. James Graham

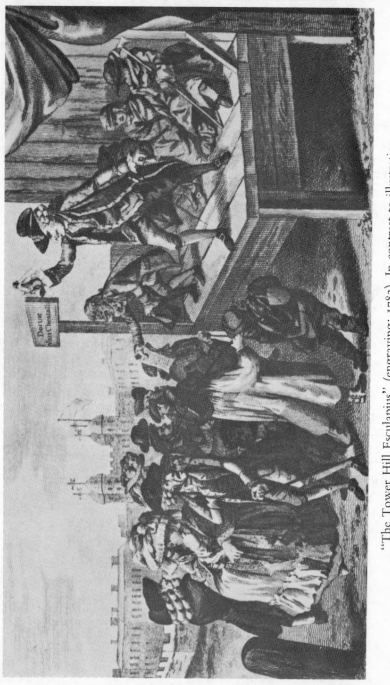

"The Tower Hill Esculapius" (engraving: 1782). In contrast to illustration number six, this quack's clientele is almost exclusively elderly to be met if cellular therapy was to succeed clinically. Firstly he postulated that only those cells which the body actively needed would be accepted by it. Any others injected disintegrated and were absorbed. Contra-indications were gradually enumerated as well. If a septic focus existed in the body, for instance a dental abscess, cells were usually rejected, Niehans argued, and rejuvenation did not recur. Radioactive Spas must be avoided and sun-bathing was prohibited after treatment. Hot baths were considered unwise, and only the minimum necessary medication with drugs was allowed. A patient in heart failure would, for instance, be allowed to continue with digitalis, but drugs like codeine and aspirin were forbidden. Finally, smoking and alcohol were interdicted.

Before Niehans decides to treat a patient by cell therapy a careful routine is insisted upon. First of all a full medical history and examination is carried out. Then a special test, the "defence ferment reaction" of Professor Emile Abderhalden, is conducted. The details of this test, carried out on the patients, is as follows:

When the functioning of an endocrine gland or of an organ is disturbed, ferments of a proteinase type appear in the blood and the urine. These ferments are absolutely specific for each gland or organ: they may be shown up by causing them to act on the albumin taken from the different glands and organs. Thus a mal-functioning of the thyroid gland will produce a "proteinase" in the blood and urine, which hydrolyses "in vitro" the albumin of the thyroid gland but affects in no way, for example, the albumins of the hypophysis, liver or brain.

The Abderhalden reaction depends on the appearing of these specific ferments. These ferments are, first of all, extracted from the urine by a process of adsorption, then they are allowed to act on the albumins of the different organs or glands for 16 hours at a temperature of 37 deg. C. and at ph. −7. If proteinases are present in the urine, they change the insoluble albumin present in the water and transform it into soluble combinations, peptons, polypepteds and amino-acids. In their turn these altered products (of the albuminous molecule) are shown up by the most varied methods, such as those which determine the total nitrogen, amino-nitrogen, or else by colorimetric methods, of which the most sensitive is the ninhydrin reaction, which stains a violet colour the product of disintegration of the albuminous molecule of the organ in question. According to the intensity of the staining obtained and according to the indications of a control scale it is possible to distinguish a strongly positive reaction (= 3), a medium positive reaction, (= 2), a slightly positive reaction, (= 1), or on the contrary, a negative reaction, (= 0). This indicates, therefore, strong, medium or slight disintegration of the albuminous molecule of the organ under examination, which, in its turn, gives a more or less parallel and proportional estimation of the functional disturbance. The normal functioning of a gland or its absence is therefore characterised by the absence of the defence ferment: its albumin suffers no change.

It must be stressed that this test is complicated and possibly obscure in its biochemistry. Apparently it can be carried out efficiently only in a few European laboratories.

Having decided that he can either treat a specific organ deficiency or carry out a positive rejuvenation Niehans admits his patients to the clinic. By means of the interpretation of the Abderhalden test, certain cells are selected for injection. These come from a variety of tissues, usually embryonic, and from many animals. Almost all the tissues of the sheep's foetus are used for various purposes. The placenta of the sheep, the hypothalamus, hypophysis and parathyroid of the calf, the testes of the young bull and the ovarian follicles, corpus luteum and suprarenals of the pig are also used.

Niehans finds that the most effective rejuvenation effects are brought about in cases of cardiac decompensation, arteriosclerosis, cerebral sclerosis, depression, diminished libido and impotence, hypertrophy of the prostate, nervous disease and hypertension.

The actual cell injections are given either personally by Niehans at the Montrose Clinic or by certain of his assistants. The technique employed is by the deep intramuscular route into the gluteus maximum muscle. When more than one type of cell is injected each nidus of injection must be placed in a fresh site in the muscle and delivered from a separate syringe. "Nature has arranged the organs in our bodies separate from each other, therefore cell suspensions of different organs should not be mixed in the same injection."[72]

Whenever possible, Niehans prefers to use fresh cells and the way these are prepared for injection is extremely important. The choice of the individual animals that will be used to obtain the donor cells is left to an experienced veterinary surgeon. Before these animals are sacrificed blood tests must demonstrate the absence of brucellosis, salmonella infection, listeriosis, leptospirosis, taxoplasmosis, and "Queensland fever". A satisfactory tuberculin reaction is also required. Niehans insists that the animals he uses are kept in a nearby *abattoir* under the direct and continuous inspection of a veterinary surgeon.

Naturally all this is very expensive. It is impossible to find out the current fees that Niehans expects for his services but a minimum bill for treatment in 1958 came to 500 Swiss francs. A breakdown of this fee showed that nearly 400 francs was set against purchase, transportation, zoological upkeep and laboratory expenses for the experimental animal. But medical, veterinary and maintenance costs really are only partly involved in the expense of Niehans cellular rejuvenation. Clinical investigation and hospitalization, so necessary Niehans feels, if a good result is to be expected, are liable to exclude anyone who does not enjoy a high income. Eight years ago the total "bill" might well reach 4,000 Swiss francs, that is roughly 1033 dollars, or £430. Present-day costs might well be treble this figure.

The removal of the selected organs which are to be used for injection from a suitably stunned but otherwise unanaesthetized animal is usually carried out by Niehans himself. When foetal tissues are required the pregnant uterus is removed *in toto*. The various tissues are then put into sterile containers and rushed to the Niehans laboratory. Waiting there is a staff of laboratory assistants who prepare individual tissues for injection by meticulous slicing and chopping by hand in Ringers solution or physiological saline.

Niehans believes that body tissues must be handled as gently as possible to retain their viability. Mechanical contrivances are therefore not used. As soon as the cell suspensions are fine enough to pass through the needle of a wide bore injection syringe, they are rushed to the bedside of the patient and injected.

The initial physical reactions to cellular therapy are very mild. Sometimes transient urticaria develops, but this soon subsides with antihistamine therapy which, apparently, Niehans feels quite justified in using, despite his "no drugs" rule. Rarely an abscess develops at the injection site. The dreaded anaphylactic reaction due to the injection of foreign protein, that most medical men would anticipate, just does not occur. After therapy patients have to lie on their faces for a short period and then have three days' complete bed rest. No long journeys are allowed for twelve days after rejuvenation, although short trips are permitted after seven days. Drugs, alcohol and tobacco are interdicted for at least three months.

Although Niehans seems to prefer fresh cell injection to bring about his rather startling rejuvenation, he has recently advocated other more convenient methods. Since 1949 he has experimented with cellular deep freezing. Tissues are removed under the same conditions as for fresh cell rejuvenation and are then rapidly frozen to between minus seventy and minus eighty degrees centigrade. During this process all the water content of the cells is removed and the powdered tissue is placed in sterile ampoules for injection. Before the injections are carried out the cells are hydrated with Ringers solution. Niehans claims these *siccazellen* are active for a year, provided they are protected from sunlight.

From the point of view of science few can hold any brief for such a process if the premise is still held that live cells really bring about the rejuvenation that Niehans apparently obtains. Although the spores of certain bacteria and seeds of some plants can resist this sort of process, the manufacture of *siccazellen* seems to sound the death knell of most animal material. Although *siccazellen* are manufactured and sold widely in Switzerland, Japan and Germany, most European and American countries boycott its sales. Niehans himself believes that *siccazellen* produces virtually equivalent results to fresh cells, but prefers fresh cells for serious cases.

Incidentally, two of Niehans' most important patients are reported to have had to make do with *siccazellen*—Chancellor Adenauer, because he was fighting an election campaign while being rejuvenated, and could not spare the time for the full clinic routine, and Sir Winston Churchill, because Niehans refused to be professionally associated with him personally, due, it is alleged, to his "share in the partition of Germany".

Niehans has experimented with tissue culture in the production of material for rejuvenation, but has largely rejected the idea on the grounds that many cells so cultured develop undesirable traits when grown artificially.

Curiously, perhaps, Niehans makes no specific claims to understand in any detail exactly how his unique method of rejuvenation works.

He admits, however, to three broad hypotheses. First of all he feels it is possible that cells injected into the muscles remain alive and migrate towards the organs that need them. He also feels it is reasonable to accept such a state of affairs because of the mobility of other wandering cells throughout the body. Secondly, he accepts the possibility of the injected cells living at the injection site, being nourished there by the host's circulation and activating the deficiencies of degenerated organs at a distance. Niehans feels this is no more unreasonable than accepting that an intramuscular injection of penicillin, given, for instance, in the thigh, will affect the tissues of the lung in a case of pneumonia.

Finally, Paul Niehans argues that even if the cells injected are attacked by the body's normal defence reactions, they may still be able to effect rejuvenation before they are destroyed.

Niehans' rejuvenation techniques have always been very strongly attacked by the Establishment in Medicine. Most doctors feel his ideas to be quite outside accepted scientific belief. Frequently, however, it would appear that prejudice rather than objectivity has been the reason for the rejection, out of hand, of Niehans' ideas.

One example is an episode that happened after Niehans had lectured at a Therapeutic Congress in Karlsruhe, in which he gave details of his technique to the medical profession. Professor Hans Schmidt of the University of Marburg visited Niehans at his house on the shores of Lake Geneva afterwards to warn him of the dangerous effects that the injection of cells could have on the body. Niehans offered to let Professor Schmidt be present at his next rejuvenation session. Reluctantly Schmidt agreed and when the moment arrived it was, apparently, a tense one, for just as Niehans was about to inject the cells into his patient the Professor took him by the arm and said, "You have already got one leg in prison: don't drag the other in after it". Niehans, however, was confident enough, having already carried out 3,000 such injections without mishap, and so he quietly completed his work. Although the minutes passed slowly after the treatment had been completed there were no untoward results. Eventually, when Professor Schmidt made his farewells to Niehans, he admitted somewhat ruefully, and referring to his own studies on anaphylactic shock, "Niehans, with one experiment you have wiped out twenty years of my life's work".[74] Later Professor Schmidt wrote a preface to Niehans' book on Cellular Therapy.

Probably the most violent objection raised by the medical profession to Niehans' work concerns the viability of the cells he injects. Although Niehans has said (see above), that the bio-logical integrity of the injected cells is not absolutely vital for rejuvenation, this remains the principal stumbling-block for general acceptance of Niehans' ideas. It is curious that one of the most damaging campaigns against Niehans was engendered, however, not on these premises but that the injected cells might multiply within the organism and produce malignant disease, for instance cancer. Niehans tried to reply to these criticisms by culturing live malignant cells and freshly removed organ cells together. Although there appeared to be no demonstrable effect between the two, and Niehans published this fact, a severe question mark had been put into men's minds and for some time no further patients applied to Niehans for treatment.

Niehans tried to regain his lost clientele by using only strains of animals that appeared to be remarkably cancer resistant. For instance, he discovered a flock of sheep in Australia some 40,000 strong that had never developed a single case of cancer according to local veterinary surgeons. But the public were unimpressed and the rejuvenator's practice temporarily languished.

Then on 12th February, 1954, Niehans was telephoned from the Vatican and requested to travel to Castel Gandolfo, where the Pope was ill. His chief physician, Dr. Galeazzi-Lizzi, was of the opinion that the Pontiff was dying of a haematemesis secondary to a gastric carcinoma. Niehans bravely acted upon the assumption that the vomiting of blood was due merely to haemorrhagic gastritis and started routine supportive therapy. Later it would appear, although concrete evidence is understandably lacking, cellular therapy was also started. Eight weeks later Niehans returned home and the Pope took up his full duties again at the Vatican. Three months later Niehans returned to give the Pope a "booster series" of injections. The newspapers, always generous with praise when things turn out well, described Niehans as "the doctor whose cell injections have rescued the Pope from death".

Later when the Pope fell ill with complications of a diaphragmatic hernia, Niehans once again attended. The Pope recovered and underwent a third course of cellular injections in 1955.

Needless to say, the honour of treating the Pope gave tremendous help to Niehan's practice as a rejuvenator. Naturally enough he has done his best to bring lasting repute to his methods. In 1963 he sent out a circular letter to all his patients in an attempt to obtain some statistical evidence on the success of his ideas. Some 89 per cent. of the patients who replied were quite convinced they had been helped by the treatment.

But perhaps the greatest evidence in favour of a turning of the scientific mind towards Niehans and his theories was the formation of an International Association for the Study of Cellular Therapy in 1960. On the occasion of his eightieth birthday Niehans was given a copy of a book, *Zellforschung und Zellulartherapie*, written by fifteen prominent scientists, and the formation of the Society has stimulated the publication of 750 scientific papers since its inception.

In the last decade cellular therapy centres have been started in many European countries. In Britain the only medical man known to carry out the treatment, however, is Vincent Blumhart Nesfield, an octogenarian with many famous patients in his rejuvenation cache. He remains silent and medically uncommunicative, although he is still said to see patients at a Harley Street address, and practises in a nursing home in Kent.

It is impossible to pronounce any verdict on Niehans' methods of rejuvenation at this stage, but careful reading of the published work in this field of activity would seem to indicate that a promising beginning has been made. Further research may realize the possibility of giving "life to years" in a way hitherto impossible.

8

Rejuvenation by Novocaine

Rumania, although a communist people's republic, does not boast a high standard of socialized medical service. Its predominantly agricultural community and unskilled industrial workers rank among the poorest in Europe, when measured by nutritional, housing and health standards. Nevertheless, this rather backward State of a little over fifteen million citizens in the last census, has one claim to fame—that of pioneering the use of novocaine in the history of rejuvenation.

In the year 1926 Professor C. I. Parhon of Bucharest suggested the world used a new word, Ilikibiology, for a special branch of biological sciences that was to concern itself with the morphological, clinical, physical and physiological changes which organisms undergo with increasing age. He also devoted himself to the study of factors that alter the rate of ageing. He had always been convinced that ageing was a pathological condition, rather than a normal run down natural process, and that differences in ageing rates could be observed in various clinical and experimental conditions.[75]

Of course differences between biological and chronological age have long been accepted by physicians. Parhon's theory of a "film of life" that can be turned both backwards and forwards at a variable speed is true enough when looked at from certain points of view. Men and women clearly "age" at different rates throughout their lives. Certain women "age" rapidly for a few years around the menopause, while their contemporary males appear "younger" for a while. Soon, however, the process is reversed and women seem to gain over men in their apparent ageing, and reach ultimately a sound enough victory in the prize of a longer chronological life. Other variations of biological time and chronological time are obvious in certain well-known pathological conditions. For example, a child suffering from an adrenal tumour may appear biologically four years older from the point of view of physical development and the radiological "age" of his bones. After the tumour has been removed these patients quickly revert to a close proximity of their chronological age.

Professor Parhon's early work involved him in a series of experiments in which pineal gland extracts were injected into mice that showed the classical signs of senility in rodents, including alopecia, hyperkeratinization, tumours, apathy, dullness and emaciation. It is not clear from which donor source this small midbrain, pineal body was obtained for these experiments and in all probability this does not matter very much. The important result of these tests carried out in conjunction with three colleagues was that the treated mice gained weight and had an improved skin suppleness and texture after treatment, as compared with untreated control animals.

Further work in this field led to investigations in which the thyroid glands, most of the parathyroid gland and the reproductive glands were removed in rats, rabbits, guinea pigs and dogs. The endocrine deficiencies produced by these mutilations included an increased rate of ageing, a speeding-up of the "life film". Parhon drew analogies between these animal experiments and the naturally decreased thyroid function in aged men (proved by basal metabolic rate studies and iodine uptake estimations), and lowered sexual function (reflected in urinary steroid levels). An interesting sidelight on the experiments demonstrated by Parhon was the changes in connective tissues that occurred. This was noticed particularly in the physical alteration of the collagen fibres of rats' tails, in the animals with multiglandular insufficiency. Changes in collagen fibres and other connective tissue fibres are perhaps one of the most fundamental characteristics of all ageing.

Professor Parhon felt justified, therefore, in assuming from his experiments and observations that he had proved that biological ageing was in certain cases, at least, a variable process. And that it was possible to alter it by speeding or slowing the "life film". But there was no specific mention of exactly how this might be practically obtained in the case of man.

Professor Parhon's work on the pineal gland produced little reaction in the scientific world until more recent times. This gland, lying as it does, suspended in the cavity of the cranium between the two cerebral hemispheres, has long been of interest to scientists and philosophers. The ancients regarded it as the seat of the soul but as early as 1892 Otto Heubner, a German neurologist, described a tumour that destroyed the pineal gland and produced various endocrine derangements, including precocious puberty in the young male victim of the disease. More recently pineal tumour enlargements have been shown to delay sexual maturity.

Gradually biological science came around to the opinion that the pineal gland was an atavistic visual structure. Certain primitive arthropods possess a medial third eye and the pineal gland in higher animals was thought to be the vestigial remnant of this. As things turned out the pineal gland was found to have a function linked with the function of the eye inasmuch as it was related to changes in animals bound up with their exposure to light.

Exactly how this information came to be discovered is highly interesting and started with an apparently irrelevant observation made in the twenties that pineal extract blanched the skin of tadpoles, although it had no effect on human skin. Eventually in 1959, Dr. A. B. Lerner, a dermatologist at Yale University, by means of painstaking research involving some quarter of a million bovine pineal glands, separated the blanching factor and christened the substance melatonin. This discovery led to further work by Dr. Julius Axelrod of the National Institute of Mental Health's Clinical science laboratory in the US in 1960. Melatonin was shown to be elaborated in the body from a neurohormone, seratonin, by enzymic action.

Early investigators had been rather misled by the fact that calcification of the pineal gland occurs in humans around the age of puberty, and this led to the assumption that any effect the gland might have in early adolescence ceased at this time. Painstaking research by Dr. Axelrod and his colleagues on post-mortem subjects showed eventually, however, that the calcified pineal is just as active biologically as it is in earlier years and gradually more facts about this curious structure came to be known. These linked up in an unexpected way with work carried out by the British endocrinologist, W. C. Rowan, some forty years previously.

Rowan had demonstrated that the annual period of testicular growth in the Junco finch could be advanced by increasing the length of time each day that birds were exposed to light. In other words, the duration of light stimuli impinging upon an animal's eye was capable of bringing about, by endocrine means, changes in the sex organs. Gradually, during more recent years, many other mysteries of the pineal gland have been unravelled. Groups of rats were kept in constant darkness for six days while others were maintained in constant light for the same period. Their pineal glands were then examined at autopsy. The animals kept in the light had smaller pineals and smaller quantities of the enzyme involved in melatonin production than those who had spent their time in darkness. Eventually it was demonstrated that light makes itself felt on the pineal gland through the sympathetic nervous system. By means of electron microscopy and radioactive tracing techniques a definite pineal rhythm acti-vity was also established.

Dr. Seymour S. Kety, chief of the National Institute of Mental Health's laboratory of Clinical Science, stated

> . . . there is a connection by way of the sympathetic nervous system to a possible inner clock. In the pineal this connection can be re-garded as having been detected in a "relay station". While the pres-ence of serotonin in the gland is clock-like, it has been shown in the rat that the whole rhythm stops when the sympathetic nerves leading

to the gland are cut. . . . It is a fascinating thing to consider that we have an internal clock set at approximately 24 hours. While there is no evidence that the pineal is itself our biological clock, we are very interested to know of its connection to a known regulating mechanism.[76]

Clearly Professor Parhon's researches on the pineal gland deserve to be remembered with reference to ideas on rejuvenation in the light of these more modern research facts, for if the resetting of an internal biological clock mechanism ever became possible a considerable rejuvenation as far as chronological age is concerned would certainly become feasible.

Research in Bucharest, however, moved away from pineal studies but nevertheless, the year 1947 was an important year for Rumanians. King Michael was forced to abdicate and the People's Republic was proclaimed. Quite soon a State scientific programme was under way and featured among its objects was research in ageing carried out at the Geriatric Centre of Bucharest, now called the C. I. Parhon Institute of Geriatrics.

In 1951 various problems of gerontology, geriatrics and iliki-biology were further explored. One hundred and eighty-nine inmates of the institute were examined carefully from the clinical and biochemical point of view, and then subjected to treatments with tissue extracts (spleen, placenta, adrenal, pineal gland, thyroid), vitamin E and balaneotherapy.

By now a new name crops up in scientific papers published from the Parhon Institute, that of Professor Aslan, who added a further therapeutic method to the battery of treatments being given at the Institute. This was offered to some of the most seriously disabled patients suffering from hypertension, degenerative joint disease, rheumatism, cirrhosis and various degenerative lesions of the nervous system. The ages of the patients varied from sixty to ninety-two. To the apparent amazement of the world, tremendous rejuvenation of these geriatric cripples occurred and Dr. Anna Aslan became, almost overnight, a *nova* in the firmament of rejuvenation.

Dr. Aslan had previously been involved in research projects in conjunction with Professor D. Danielopolu, and at her own clinic in Timisoara, which involved the treatment of asthma, arthritis and limb embolism with novocaine. Later this was extended to cover the treatment of achrocyanosis and trophic ulcers. One of the difficulties in the assessment of this work is the impossibility of coming to any definite scientific conclusions, due to the absence of anything remotely like a controlled clinical trial being set up at any stage, from which relevant statistical evidence might emerge. In the case of arthritis, however, the published work does give some evidence of an approximation at the very least to accepted principles of experimental medicine.

Arthritis was induced experimentally among animals by means of formaldehyde injections, and later treated by intra-arterial injection of novocaine solutions. Surprisingly an effective healing took place. What is more, animals receiving novocaine therapy showed an increased resistance to further attempts to produce arthritis by experiment. During these experiments Aslan noticed "special effects on the general state of nutrition of the treated animals, increase in weight, development of shiny fur . . . This caused us to ascribe this substance general trophic effects".[77]

Influenced perhaps by these interesting results, in the early 1950s Dr. Aslan started a relatively large number of people, forty-five in-patients in the Institute's hospital, and 2,500 out-patients, on intramuscular injections of 5 millilitres of a 2 per cent solution of novocaine (at a ph of 4.2 to 5), three times weekly, for an indefinite and varying period. Although no statistics are given as to how many patients benefited from the treatment, individual case history reports are remarkable.

V.V. was an old, inactive, weak and senile woman in 1949, as well she might be at the age of ninety-one. She had been under observation for some seven years and suffered from many symptoms of senility, including urinary incontinence, poor muscle tone, pruritis, seriously impaired hearing and vision and hypertension. From the description of her clinical condition she clearly also suffered from osteoporosis, early senile dementia and arthritis.

After the first course of novocaine therapy her arthritic and osteoporotic pain disappeared and her general condition improved. Two years later, after more treatment, the pruritis got better, her hearing became more acute and the condition of the skin was much improved. Later in the same year her muscles were stronger, she walked well and could even touch the floor with her fingers while bending from the waist. During the next year her hair, which had previously been white, started to grow darker at the temples. She was also able to concentrate better. By 1956, when she was ninety-seven, the hair growth was 80 per cent of its former dark colour, she was generally lively, managed to climb the Institute stairs, went out by herself and was able to talk sensibly about new and past experiences. She weighed four and a half kilos more than she did when treatment was commenced.

Another case, this time a seventy-year-old resident of the clinic, initially suffered from glaucoma, cataract, arteriosclerosis, arthritis and depressive illness. Her skin was atrophied and keratotic and her hair grey. In 1952 she had a stroke and it was decided to treat this with intravenous novocaine, twice daily, followed by a course of intramuscular novocaine. As might be expected she gradually recovered from the hemiplegia resultant upon the stroke. It is interesting to record that although she was initially comatose after her stroke she regained consciousness for about ten minutes after each intravenous novocaine injection.

Her subsequent progress would seem to be truly remarkable. One year after her stroke she had gained two kilograms in weight, the condition of her skin was better and she was lively and optimistic. Her muscular power as measured by the dynamometer was improved and her hair was completely repigmented.

Anyone who has visited the psychogeriatric wards of a mental hospital would be familiar with the general description of a third case described by Dr. Aslan, and would probably despair at any likelihood of rejuvenation or rehabilitation.

T.J. was a man of sixty-six. The diagnosis was post-psychic aphasia, amnesia and premature senility. He was wasted, could not remember names, manage any continuity of thought or even dress himself. There were signs of Parkinsonism and he had a "sad, frightened look, much loss of hair, partial greying and a lack of orientation". Treatment with male hormones and Vitamin B1 brought about no improvement but a lengthy course of novocaine (ten courses of twelve injections), effected a tremendous change. The depression lifted, he was able to converse and absorb new facts. He gained 4.5 kilograms in weight, his performance on the dynamometer improved and the vital capacity of his chest became greater.

It would probably not add very much to the case for novocaine rejuvenation to elaborate on further case histories. From the scientific point of view it is possible to pick fairly large holes in most of them, and perhaps the greatest criticism is that all the patients involved come under the influence of Dr. Aslan, and under the therapeutic wing of the clinic at roughly the same time as their novocaine therapy started. Nevertheless, there are certain aspects of these cases that cannot be satisfactorily explained on the grounds of psychotherapy or nutritional science any more than they can solely on the grounds of fairly prolonged novocaine therapy.

First of all the increase in hair-growth and pigmentation is remarkable. The improvement of the depressive features, without the use of modern psychotherapeutic drugs is quite amazing as well. Although good, well-planned physiotherapy might help the elderly profoundly, no physiotherapist would give much for her chances of getting a ninety-one-year-old and virtually bedridden arthritic to the stage that she could go about herself and climb stairs at the age of ninety-eight.

Dr. Aslan's studies were not confined only to the general aspects of ageing. Degenerative diseases of joints are extremely common among the elderly and are also perhaps some of the most difficult of all presenile conditions to treat effectively. Nevertheless, a series of one hundred old people with such disabilities did well, provided that continuous therapy was maintained. It is unlikely that any patients would improve with no treatment, but the possibility of a placebo response cannot be excluded in this series of patients, twenty-six of whom showed considerable improvement and only fourteen no improvement at all.

Novocaine therapy was finally extended by Aslan to prophyl-axis and a regimen instigated to prevent ageing. It was suggested that this might well start at the age of forty, a series of twelve injections being given over the first prophylactic month, and then repeated every other, or every third month. By 1957 well over five thousand patients were so treated.

Dr. Aslan has repeatedly been accused of not publishing statistical results, and to some extent this criticism is justified. Some statistics have been made known however. Taking a total of 1,370 patients admitted to the Institute between 1953 and 1957, of whom 875 were treated with novocaine and the rest by "other biotrophic" means, that are unspecified, her results are significant. The death rate of the novocaine group was 2.7 per cent and the "control" group 10.3 per cent.

A smaller group of out-patients examined showed similar results. In those treated with novocaine the death rate was nearly 8 per cent (average age of death eighty-three years), while the death rate of the controls, defined as those who only "had drugs suited to disease" was about 42 per cent. The rehabilitation rate on novocaine therapy was also impressive, nearly twice as many patients were pronounced fit for work in the novocaine group as in the "normal treatment" group.

The world in general has not judged the Aslan rejuvenation technique with any great kindness or interest. Typical of Western reaction was a leading article of the *British Medical Journal*.[78] For reasons that will be explained later, Aslan eventually chris-tened her novocaine solution "H3" and the mystery of this short-hand title captured the imagination of the Press. Typical of the reactions was that of Hugh McLeave's article in the London *Daily Mail*, which told of the six centenarians under Aslan's care at Bucharest all of whom were active and agile, one being able to perform the remarkable feat of "hand-balancing" on the floor without showing any signs of physical exertion or distress.[79]

Such material being published always seems to incite disfavour in the breast of the medical Establishment, particularly as some doctors, believing that H3 was a mysterious new therapeutic substance, had clamoured for its "release" as a drug in this country. The plain statement that it was simply a 2 per cent solution of procaine, at a *ph* of between 4.2 and 5 per cent (procaine is the British N.F. official name for novocaine), something, incidentally, never in any way denied by the workers at the Parhon Institute, clearly upset British medical opinion.

The *British Medical Journal* leader also stressed that procaine is broken down in a few minutes by the procaine esterase of the plasma, and to a lesser extent by a liver enzyme, into aminobenzoic acid and diethylamino-ethanol, information originally made widely known by Dr. Aslan some three years previously. It also stressed that this substance was entirely eliminated from the blood stream within twenty minutes. It also pointed out in the *Journal* that it was "difficult to understand the system of dosage, especially as Professor Aslan admits that similar results cannot be obtained by the break-down products of procaine".

About a week before the *British Medical Journal* leader was published, Professor Aslan had given a lecture at London's ancient Apothecaries' Hall on "Procaine therapy in old age, and other Trophic Disturbances". This lecture could hardly have been less of a success. To begin with, it was sponsored by the *Daily Mail*, who unfortunately thought it necessary to make an ill-advised announcement that Dr. Aslan's lecture was to be considered confidential and not communicated in any way to the (rival) National Press. The special correspondent of the *British Medical Journal* who reported the proceedings clearly formed a poor opinion of the meeting. A subtle slight on the audience may not have been intended in the remark that those present were "mainly general practitioners". Then at the last minute the chairman did not appear and a deputy was hurriedly appointed.

Unfortunately at her lecture, Professor Aslan experienced language difficulties, but managed to preface her remarks with a tribute in English to British achievements in geriatrics before briefly outlining the background of her work in excellent French. Later she handed her manuscript to a translator who read it in English. But no new facts came to light and when the paper was finished the audience were invited to pose any questions they might have on procaine rejuvenation. Unhappily as far as our subject is concerned the special correspondent's report was a disappointment as "none of these questions, or Dr. Aslan's replies to them added greatly to what she had already said".

The *British Medical Journal's* account of the meeting deplored the clinical reports of the Parhon Group. Presumably this referred to the publications issued previously by the Parhon Institute of Geriatrics.[80] They made, it said, "sad reading for the clinician trained in modern scientific methods. There is an almost complete absence of controls, and blind trials were never used". A careful perusal of the relevant papers, however, hardly substantiates the complete absence of controls, although admittedly there were no blind trials.

Blind trials, in which no one involved knows which patients are being treated with the method being investigated—patient, nurse, staff or doctor, are, of course, not justifiably applicable to all forms of medical research. If, for instance, a reasonably well substantiated cure for inoperable or otherwise incurable cancer were to come to light in which it appeared on clinical grounds that large numbers of patients were possibly being prevented from dying due to the exhibition of a new drug or treatment, it is doubtful that any clinician, even if trained in the "modern scientific method", would feel justified in withholding it from his dying patients. Professor Aslan may well have looked at her geriatric patients in the same way if she was convinced that to withhold therapy was to condemn so many to a premature grave.

Another assertion that damages Professor Aslan's reputation also sprang from the same *British Medical Journal* report. Although it went on to say "Professor Aslan created a most favourable personal impression as a woman gifted with humour, charm and enthusiasm and [here was the rub], boundless therapeutic optimism . . . there is no real evidence that it [procaine] is any good at all, and the extensive publicity given it in the Press will have the unfortunate effect of raising the hopes of many that at last the Elixir of Life has been discovered. The search for this, for the philosopher's stone, for the panacea, makes a fascinating chapter in the history of healing: and has always turned out to be the dream child of the chemist".

In all probability the resistance felt by the medical profession to procaine rejuvenation sprang from three main causes. First, the sensational newspaper reports that seem to plague even the slightest whisper in medical literature of the word rejuvenation. Then there was the fact that the work done on procaine rejuvenation hailed from behind the Iron Curtain. British and American opinion is deeply suspicious of medical reports that hail even from certain European countries. To accept reports coming from Rumania at this time seemed almost to smack of therapeutic nihilism. Some people obviously thought Dr. Aslan to be a rogue presenting her cases cleverly selected to gain some world-wide reputation in rejuvenation. Others clearly labelled her a charming example of the scientific self-deceptionist.

But the main reason for the rejection of novocaine rejuvenation stemmed from none of these rather odd psychological suspicions. What seemed most baffling was that there was no logical explanation as to how procaine rejuvenation could work. The main stumbling-block was the extremely rapid breakdown of procaine in the bloodstream into two relatively inert chemical substances. How could this, under any circumstances, be held responsible for any rejuvenating property?

Professor Aslan's published work is always very guarded with reference to the biochemistry of novocaine. She stands by her expressed opinion that old age is a dystrophy, and that the observed progressive degeneration of the elderly can be checked by novocaine. Experiments carried out and the rates of growth of certain bacterial and infusorial colonies of organisms in the laboratory have strengthened her conviction that novocaine and its breakdown products have a vitamin-like or biocatalytic property. The rather mysterious H_3 item that crept into the nomenclature of rejuvenation was merely a shorthand expression coined by Aslan to differentiate novocaine from its breakdown products. On the whole she believes that the fundamental effect of novocaine may be at the level of cellular oxidation-reduction levels.

The fact that novocaine is quickly broken down into substances in the body that have little or no rejuvenating action has never been denied by Aslan. But to deny that novocaine therapy à la Aslan has no physical effect is to deny many of the published facts, or to enclose them in a terrific package deal of scientific fraud designed presumably to confuse the Western world.

For instance, experiments carried out at the Berkovitza farm in Bulgaria showed that lambs treated over a thirty-day period with novocaine increased in weight to the extent of nearly 15 per cent against those of a control group. Oscillometric tests in elderly men, combined with local and general stress studies were carried out and a relationship was demonstrated between oscillograph tracings and arterial tonus, elasticity and reactivity. While the results of these investigations showed a gradual degeneration of arterial function over the years in untreated patients, novocaine therapy produced a reversal of this trend. In other experiments the circulation time was taken as a rough and ready index of vascular adaptability and this, under normal circumstances, increased with age. But this also returns to early chronological values after novocaine treatment. Another and little-understood biochemical observation is that changes in the relative proportions of albumin to globulin in the blood could be profoundly effected by novocaine therapy.

Other physiological effects of an inexplicable nature have also been published. In one scientific paper that studied the intravenous injection of a single injection of novocaine it was found that the number of circulating white cells increases significantly in the second hour after injection.[81]

One of the ultimate tests that scientific minds look for whenever an apparent breakthrough is postulated is whether the results claimed can be confirmed by other skilled workers in the same field of study. As far as novocaine therapy has been concerned there is little evidence that anyone has repeated Aslan's remarkable work. The nearest published report that would seem to substantiate her claims comes from Germany, where two physicians carried out a series of novocaine injections on the inhabitants of the old-age home in the City of Halle.[82] One or two series of injections were given, and the results were encouraging as far as arteriosclerotic and arthritic complaints were concerned. Later tests included the simultaneous injection of a multivitamin preparation as well as novocaine, and so results can hardly be said to have been comparable. The authors, however, were cagey about using the term rejuvenation. Perhaps the realization that they were dealing with verbal dynamite as far as the reception of their paper was concerned acted as sufficient warning.

In this country no one seems seriously interested in proving or disproving Aslan's work. Dr. Abraham Marcus, the *Sunday Observer's* medical correspondent, quoted one small clinical trial carried out by a Yorkshire geriatrician that was designed to test the therapy in such a way as to be acceptable to the British medical opinion. The results as far as rejuvenation was concerned were entirely negative. Significantly, however, in the history of ideas on this subject, it was the admitted fact that improvement on hair and skin characteristics occurred. In the US on the whole there is little or no interest shown apart from one important clinical trial that was carried out at the Patton State Hospital in California.

This took the form of a small but well-organized double blind therapeutic trial. Forty-five patients were selected for the survey, each seventy years or older. They all had a history of arteriosclerosis and degenerative arthritis. They also had fairly well developed organic mental deterioration with symptoms that included memory defects and a general clouding of the sensorium. For instance, only six of the patients knew what the time was, fourteen knew where they were. Thirteen knew who they were. Twenty-eight could remember where they were born but only ten knew who was President of the US. All had been in the mental hospital for ninety days but none more than five years.

These forty-five patients were then divided up into three groups of fifteen. Each of these groups received a series of injections three times a week for a total of ten doses. Then, after a rest period of one week, a second course of ten injections was given. The injections given all appeared similar and no one involved in the trial knew "who" was getting "which" injection. In actual fact one injection was procaine, one a mixture of vitamin B1 and nicotinic acid and the other a solution of *normal* saline.

Not all the patients completed the trial. One died, two sustained fracture of the hip and were transferred to other wards, one had to be removed from the trial due to violence and two others developed episodes of acute illness. This reduced the test patients to thirty-nine.

After the trial the patients were critically examined with reference to improvement in their physical and psychiatric condition, together with a battery of laboratory tests similar to those they had received before the trial. The results were highly interesting. First of all there was "no discernible improvement or deterioration revealed attributable to the injections of procaine". This might well be thought to spell the death knell of procaine rejuvenation were it not for the following points.

First, in any clinical trial including double blind surveys, there is a procedural effect (placebo response) that is usually quite predictable. In this case it was absent. The organizers felt that this was due to the "method used", for the patients, it was claimed, did not receive any additional attention as a result of partaking in the trial. This would seem to be an invalid argument when one considers the formidable selection procedure of the patients involved, their initial assessment, the laboratory tests, the injections themselves and then the post "rejuvenation" medical examination with more tests.

Another point worth stressing relative to this particular clinical trial is that it was not continued for long enough to be strictly comparable with Aslan techniques. But this palls beside what appears to be the most serious criticism and that is that the patients selected were rather too far advanced in their general physical and mental deterioration to be considered fit for any rejuvenation method. The fact that six out of forty-five fell by the wayside for various medical reasons during the brief trial would seem to support this basic criticism.[83] In all probability the trial failed to show any response for the same reason that there was no placebo response, the patients involved were confused and deteriorated creatures beyond the help of any medical aid.

Professor Aslan, like many rejuvenators, believes in taking her own medicine. Those who know her remark on her apparent lack of years and her lively mentality.

It is curious, perhaps, that procaine, this time mixed with caffeine, is the basis of another idea in the history of rejuvenation. Dr. Huneke of Dusseldorf uses it as the basis for rejuvenating and other treatments as part of the medical credo that he calls neural therapy. It is interesting to contrast the careful, plodding, institutional and long-term techniques used at the Parhon Geriatric Centre with the queues of patients Huneke treats in his consulting rooms. Dr. Richard MacKarness, who interviewed Dr. Huneke recently (personal communication), had the opportunity of watching his technique at close quarters. He felt that he had a brusque, almost Prussian presence, and bullied his patients; an unusual guise in which to find a professional rejuvenator. Huneke examines his patients for evidence of previous inflammations or common sites of infection. Commonly he finds this in the base of the teeth or in the tonsillar area. In other cases he turns his attention to old scars anywhere on the body. In these areas he injects a solution of novocaine and caffeine.

Apparently in about 20 per cent of cases there is an instant reaction to Huneke's injection of a very favourable nature. Crippling arthritis suddenly becomes painless or a stoop straightens. The doctor refers to this as the *secunden phenomenam* (flash phenomenon), that cures. Although the British and American orthodox medicine have no time for this curious technique, Huneke's defence is that it works, and the crowds who flock for treatment by neural therapy are tangible testimonials to his success.

Huneke says of his technique, "the nervous system from its central parts, the brain and the spinal cord, sends ramifications into every corner of the body, so that all organs are interconnected with nervous pathways. Irritation at any point in the nervous system distorts the harmonious working of the body and can encourage pain and inflammation everywhere". Few thinking people would agree that this idea in the history of rejuvenation warrants very much serious study, although Huneke proudly claims he can cure half the world's chronic sick by means of his "conservative knife", as one enthusiastic French professor referred to his long-needled syringe, and hundreds of German doctors have attended Huneke's clinical demonstrations to watch him in action.

9

The Sex Glands and Rejuvenation

In all probability there is no story in the history of medicine more complicated with reference to facts and fallacy, more disappointing measured in high hopes that finished up as profound disappointments, and more poignant with regard to fine reputations dashed on the rocks of vindictive criticism, than that of the sex glands and the part they have played in the history of ideas on rejuvenation.

The beginning of this story starts logically with Charles Edouard Brown-Séquard, who was born in the year 1817 in the then British island of Mauritius. Son of an Irish-American sea captain and a French woman from the nearby island Reunion, he graduated as a doctor in Paris at the age of twenty-three and returned to his native home with the intention of practising medicine there. A facet of Brown-Séquard's character was, however, an intractable professional wanderlust, and very soon his interest in experimental medicine led him to Harvard. A few years later he left the US to take up the Chair of Comparative Medicine in Paris, only to migrate to England in 1859 when he became Physician to the National Hospital for the Paralysed and the Epileptic, as it was then called, in Queen's Square, London. Five years later the physician was back at Harvard as Professor of Physiology and Nervous Diseases. Never seeming able to stay more than a few years in one place, Brown-Séquard subsequently returned to

Paris for a few years as Professor at the Ecole de Médicine. Yet again he returned to New York but then came back to Paris to succeed the great neurologist Claude Bernard, as Professor of Experimental Medicine, in the Collège de France in 1878, a position he held until his death on 2nd April, 1894.

Although Brown-Séquard's life seems a little unsettled academically it was, of course, a very successful one especially from the point of view of medical research. He confirmed Claude Bernard's work on the sympathetic nervous system, provided valuable knowledge of the effects of arrangement of the nerve fibres in the spinal cord, conducted important experimental work on the subject of epilepsy as well as studies on heat exhaustion and the nervous system generally. He also had the distinction of founding and editing two learned medical journals. The *Journal de la physiologie de l'homme et des animaux*, which ran from 1858 to 1863, and the *Archives de physiologie normale et pathologique* which was founded in 1868 and produced until Brown-Séquard died.

All things considered, Brown-Séquard's life, although rather unusual for his time and somewhat irregular in several ways, was one of busy professionalism. It has been stated that he produced around five hundred scientific papers and essays during his lifetime. Naturally some of his experimental work has subsequently been discredited, notably that relative to the distribution of anaesthesia following hemiplegia.[84] Brown-Séquard has also been criticized about certain experiments in which he claimed to have shown that the progeny of animals in which he had induced epilepsy artificially, themselves developed epilepsy. Another apparent flaw in his experimental methods would seem to be demonstrated by what can only be described as an observation that otherwise supports the fallacy of maternal impressions.

Once again in the pursuance of research on experimental epilepsy Brown-Séquard carried out sections of the sciatic nerve in certain guinea pigs. Probably as a result of the anaesthesia of the leg produced by the operation, certain of these animals tended to bite and even nibble off certain parts of their numb toes and legs. Although Brown-Séquard had been breeding guinea pigs for thirty years in his various laboratories he had never observed a single case of toeless guinea pigs, yet in thirteen cases toeless progeny were born to the parent animals whose sciatic nerves had been sectioned.[85]

These extraordinary experimental results have never been confirmed by other workers, and in all probability other explanations existed for these curious teratogenetic effects. However, they do not in any way detract from the mass of the great experimental physiologist's scientific work that remained entirely untarnished until 1889 when an event occurred that was to lead to the downfall of Brown-Séquard's professional reputation.

For several years previously he had been in the habit of carrying out personal dynamometer tests, presumably to observe experimentally the effects of age. As he approached seventy he was able to record the onset of muscular decline. As it happened, during the next two or three years, Brown-Séquard also suffered from fibrositis, pronounced fatigue and sleeplessness.[86] Some time during the spring of 1889 he had been experimenting with extracts made from various endocrine glands, and most likely this was an extension of previous work published between 1856 and 1858 that demonstrated an "Addison disease like syndrome" in animals in which the supradrenal glands had been removed.

This eventually led Brown-Séquard to experiment upon himself, injecting extracts made from the testes of guinea pigs. The results were apparently startling, for he found himself surprisingly rejuvenated, not only sexually but also as far as muscular power, demonstrated on the dynamometer, was concerned. On 1st June, 1889, remembered by some as the birthday of the theory of internal secretion and the science of endocrinology,[87] the professor made a statement at a meeting of the Sociéte de Biologie that was world-shattering in its conception. Holding a small phial of fluid in his hand for all to see, he disclosed that he had made an extract of animal sexual glands and that although he had had only three injections of it so far he was tremendously rejuvenated. Brown-Séquard had married recently, for the third time, and was indiscreet enough to boast to the assembled audience that he had been able to *rendre visite* to the young Madame Brown-Séquard after the injections. This added spice and sensationalism to a meeting that had gathered presumably to hear a cold and serious scientific paper.

Brown-Séquard must have looked as he alleged he felt, thirty years younger, for the popular French papers jumped on the news with alacrity. *Le Matin* immediately opened a subscription to erect an Institute of Rejuvenation where the *Méthode Séquardienne* was to be practised for the benefit of senescent Frenchmen. Brown-Séquard and his assistant, D'Arsonval, invented "a fantastic Rube Goldberg type of machine with a belt pulley, tubes, alembics, aeration bladders, instrument dials: into it he fed bull testes, pulped, filtered through sand, ascepticized with boric acid, drawn off as a liquor . . . to be pumped into the gluteus maximus of thousands of aged but still libidinous boulevardiers".[33]

Quite soon, however, Brown-Séquard found there were vociferous critics willing to crucify him and his ideas. One German newspaper retorted promptly, "Professor Brown-Séquard's audience appears to have received an impression of the intellectual capacity of the aged scientist very different from that which he in his elevated frame of mind evidently expected to produce. The lecture must be regarded as further proof for the necessity of retiring professors who have attained their three score years and ten".[88]

Another newspaper alleged that the professor had done little in the last few years to follow the progress of science, and dismissed his experiments as "senile aberrations". Later, when reading a paper to the Paris Academy of the Sciences, Brown-Séquard stressed "I have never contended that my method enables me to influence irreparable senile changes. . . . I hope, however, that every unprejudiced and reflective person will recognize the soundness of my conclusions as soon as he has become convinced of the accuracy of the facts and of the logical force of the demonstrations". Somewhat later Brown-Séquard claimed there was a definite aid to mental work inherent in the induction of sexual excitement, not proceeding to emission,[6] and in this perhaps we can see the first signs of his own disenchantment with rejuvenation.

It has been suggested that the method used for the mass extraction of testes by Brown-Séquard was the reason for its inefficiency.[89] There may have been some truth in this for excitement in Paris soon simmered down as far as the general public was concerned. The medical profession was never enthusiastic. From the personal point of view the débâcle of his rejuvenation methods brought tragedy to Brown-Séquard. Apart from a paper in 1892 in which he argued that the kidney produced an internal secretion, no further work was published. His young wife deserted him and he died on the Riviera of a cerebrovascular accident in 1894.

Whether or not Brown-Séquard's therapy had any physical action or not we do not know. Aqueous extracts of the testes of mammals contain testosterone and possibly other androgenic substances. Inactivation of testosterone, when it is injected, is quite rapidly carried out in the liver, and current pharmacological opinion states quite firmly that synthetic testosterone at any rate has little or no effect on senile or psychic impotence. Nor is it an effective aphrodisiac. There is, however, an anabolic effect after testosterone injection in which well known biological changes, such as nitrogen retention, and increase in body and organ weight occur and so some rejuvenating factor presumably is present.

In 1861, at the time Brown-Séquard was enjoying his rather peripatetic physiological researches around the world, a son was born to a doctor practising in the town of Hohenems in the Austrian province of Vararlberg. He was destined to become one of the best known names in the history of rejuvenation.

The life of Eugen Steinach had an inauspicious beginning. After leaving school he was sent to study medicine in Geneva, and later in Vienna, where he obtained his M.D. His interests were mainly in the field of experimental physiology and after working at the Physiological Institute of the University of Innsbruck for three years he obtained in 1890, a coveted post as first assistant to Ewald Hering in Prague. Professor Hering is remembered for producing, in 1870, a "psychophysical theory that facultative memory, the automatic power of protoplasm to do what it has done before, is the distinctive property of all living matter".[2]

The young physiologist clearly found the intellectual climate of the nineties intensely stimulating. Gone were the days of speculative natural philosophy. Natural phenomena were being investigated in the light of the newly appreciated laws of chemistry and physics. The impact of the basic bacteriological truths described by Koch, Pasteur, Löffler and Edwin Kelbs, in the previous two decades, was still very much in the minds of men of science. A mechanistic and chemical interpretation was being sought for life's vital forces.

The organic structure of man obeyed the laws of physics, ionic concentration was responsible for muscular activity, and nervous excitation, the principle of conservation of energy, a sufficient explanation for metabolic processes, and even the dynamics of the circulation was governed by physical laws... even the dark secret of sex and the sexes was believed to be initiated and dominated by mechanistic and chemical phenomena.[87]

Steinach's previous work had been devoted to the physiology of muscles and nerves, but in 1892 he came across a paper written by the neurologist, I. R. Tarchanoff, on the "physiology of the sex apparatus of the Frog", in which the sex instinct, particularly the mechanism of attraction that the female frog held for the male, was explored for the first time scientifically. Tarchanoff also suggested that the seminal vesicles, organs that become enlarged from the size of an apple pip to that of a wild strawberry during the mating season, were the prime activators of the central nervous system that trigger off the typical mating behaviour in the male frog. Initial experiments with frogs led him to believe that Tarchanoff was wrong, and Steinach decided to repeat his work using a higher order of animals, namely the Rat (*Mus decumanus*).

Steinach's early work with the rat is a fine example of straight-forward observational research and animal experiment. Strength tests were elaborated, courage reactions assessed, and it was possible to deduce that environment profoundly affected the male rat's sexual behaviour. This led Steinach to postulate psychic sexual factors being present in his laboratory animals. As a result of surgically removing the seminal vesicles of several rats he was able to prove, in 1894, that they were simply semen storage organs and had no part in the production or maintenance of sexual function.

Although John Hunter in 1762 and von Berthold in 1849 had,

by transplantation experiments in cockerels, suggested that the sex glands affected the blood, maintained the sexual characteristics and reacted on the central nervous system via the blood stream, their work was not generally accepted and Steinach's next series of experiments sought to finally establish or disprove this theory. For many scientists believed that in these earlier bird experiments complete excision of the testes was not carried out at operation. And that nervous connections between the testes and the central nervous system remained that invalidated the experiments.

Steinach, during the years between 1900 and 1910, produced a beautiful series of experiments proving conclusively that castration prevented the maturation of the sexual impulse, and that transplantation of testes from other animals could bring about sexual maturity in young castrates. He also found that castration of the matured rat did not remove all masculinity. A certain variable sexual impulse survived after castration.

Steinach postulated the existence of a psychic sexual force at work in these cases that augmented glandular factors, and he designed a series of experiments to investigate this quotient of sexuality. This took the shape of a series of tests in which young, weaned male rats were brought up either singly or in groups of four, isolated from any female influence. The introduction of these rats when they became sexually mature to female rats in heat was carried out at progressively greater intervals in their lifetime. When the interval was only of a month's duration, sexual behaviour was quite normal. When this was extended to six months, however, the sexual impulse "had sustained more or less damage". After ten or eighteen months isolation from all females, the males became completely sexually apathetic and impotent, and their secondary sex characteristics showed progressive deterioration. Post-mortem examination of such animals showed pronounced atrophic changes in the sex glands.

A further experiment showed that this psychic inhibition was also reversible. In one large compartment of a cage were placed rats rendered impotent by isolation, and in a small compartment a rutting female was introduced. Gradually, after a few days, the previously apathetic rats showed increasing activity. Normal

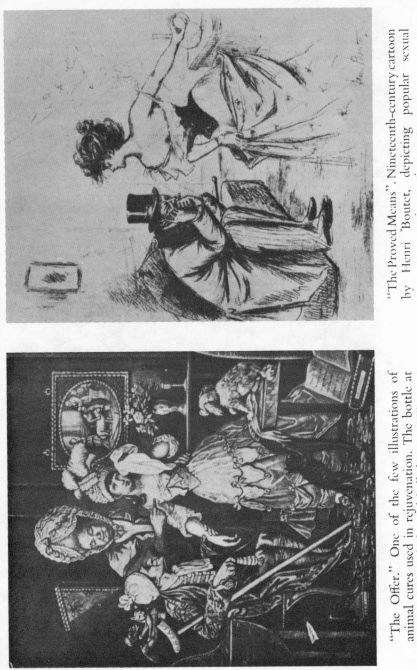

"The Offer." One of the few illustrations of animal cures used in rejuvenation. The bottle at the old man's feet is labelled Viper Wine

"The Proved Means". Nineteenth-century cartoon by Henri Boutet, depicting popular sexual rejuvenating nostrums

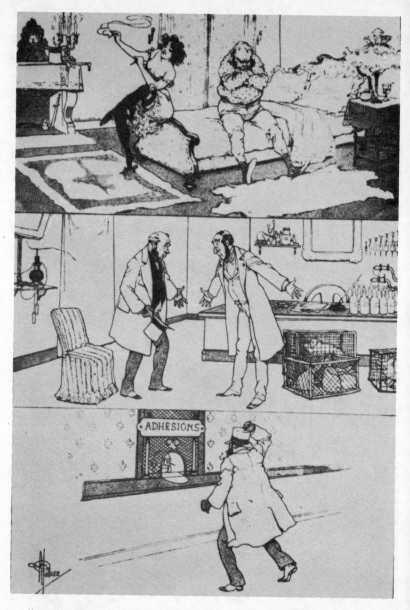

"How one becomes a member of the morality club"—a German
joke on the theme of Hobson's choice

male aggressive behaviour ensued and after two weeks, if the dividing barrier between the previous isolates and a rutting female was removed, immediate sexual activity commenced. If specimens were now examined post-mortem, the internal genitals had returned to normal size and shape.

Steinach was also able to show that in the case of rats this psychic rejuvenation was brought about in all probability via the sense of smell, for blinded isolate males were rejuvenated as easily as were sighted animals.

These neatly-arranged experiments led Steinach to believe, by the end of 1910, that the primary causal control of sex life is invested in the genital glands, but that there is in certain circumstances an overriding central nervous control. By means of further experiments in which he proved that genital-gland extracts, when injected, can produce secondary sexual changes in frogs, he finally divorced the possibility of nervous contact between the sex glands and the brain being responsible for sexual behaviourisms, as had previously been widely believed. The relationship was thus proved to be brought about by chemical or hormonal substances.

In these latter experiments Steinach was really extending to lower animals some of the claims that Brown-Séquard had made some twenty years before. As far as sexual maturation and behaviourisms were concerned he might well have felt that he had fully substantiated Brown-Séquard. By now, of course, the results of experimental work on the endocrine glands, the glands of internal secretion, were widely known to scientists throughout Europe. The mysteries of the pancreas were being unravelled. A transplantation of a particle of thyroid gland from a mother into her myxoedematous daughter had been successful. Tetany had been treated by implantation of the parathyroids of oxen, and the mysteries of the pituitary itself were beginning to be understood. It is natural enough that Steinach, now deeply involved in physiological problems should turn his attention to the effect of this organ, particularly as reports from both Europe and the US had indicated that pituitary depletion produced sexual atrophy.

By now Steinach had also explored the complex field of feminization of males and masculination of females, using guinea pigs as his experimental animals. By means of transplantation of ovaries into infantile castrated guinea pigs, he successfully demonstrated the feminization with regard to the development of breasts and nipples, milk secretion, willingness to suckle, hirsute type, skeletal form and the flowering of the female psyche was possible.[90] And subsequently that splayed female guinea pigs could be successfully masculized by means of testicular implants.[91] Two years later he showed that implantation of ovary and testes into immature male castrates produced experimental hermaphroditism.

By the time of the outbreak of the first world war, Steinach was probably the first and foremost research worker in the physiology of sex. During the war years biological work at the research Institute in Vienna, never particularly lavishly endowed with funds, lost momentum. But the only paper published during the war period by Steinach in 1916 was a highly significant one from the point of view of ideas in rejuvenation, for it demonstrated that if the ovaries of immature guinea pigs were irradiated so as to obliterate as far as possible the germinal, reproductive cells, the interstitial cells of the ovary proliferated and produced greatly accentuated secondary sexual characteristics in the animals.

After the war Steinach continued in his experiments and carried out the preliminary work that was to preoccupy him for the rest of his life and place him in the unique position from which he has probably never been ousted, that of the biologist whose researches have contributed most to the science of rejuvenation.

But even at this early stage Steinach was beginning to feel the slings and arrows that seem to be almost an occupational hazard of those who interest themselves in such subjects. He wrote:

Since the evident facts of reactivation [as Steinach referred to the results of his researches involving the puberty gland or its extract], which have now been experimentally confirmed throughout the world, defied contradiction, the opposition endeavoured to prevent the spread of knowledge and the ever-progressive work of the initiator, his co-operators and his adherents. To this end books were written, lectures delivered, numerous tracts compiled, all of which were full of misrepresentations and misunderstandings of my work, and were, accordingly apt to prejudice the general public, physicians and laymen.

Steinach was at this time hoping for an Institute to materialize worthy of his continuing researches. It did not, and eventually the small laboratory where his all-important work had been carried out had to close down due to lack of funds. The year was 1920 and Steinach felt his scientific work and aspiration doomed to failure.

Anyone who studies Steinach's work, however superficially, cannot fail to be impressed with his careful methods, the humanity with which he conducted his numerous laboratory experimental operations, and his respect for the welfare and care of the small animals with which he worked. He obviously read voraciously and was constantly in tune with the tenor of scientific advances. As might be expected, he was not long put down by the disappointment of the 1920s and was soon organizing himself in further experimental work, this time in conjunction with the Pharmaceutical Industry of Germany, for Schering Aktein-Gesellschaft, a firm to this day well known for its work in the pharmacological aspects of endocrinology, started production of sex hormones commercially and entrusted Steinach with the task of biological assay in the production of their drugs. In this way funds became available for the next step in his research programme.

It is impossible to give a date at which Steinach's mind turned more definitely towards the possibilities of the rejuvenating effects of hormones. The idea was certainly germinal in the second decade of the twentieth century, when he noted changes in temperament and physique in prematurely senescent castrated rats in which he effected puberty by means of gonad transplantation. The first real evidence, however, of a fresh driving force in Steinach's career was a paper published in 1920[92] in which he showed that senile male rats were rejuvenated by the simple process of vasoligation.

Steinach gave full details of the technique of this operation. The animals were anaesthetized by putting them in a "bell jar" with some cotton wool impregnated with ether. When they were in a "deep stupor" they were removed and the belly, groin and scrotum carefully shaved and disinfected. Should the animals show any signs of "coming round" more ether was administered on a tiny mask and the scrotum was then opened by a small incision. The vas deferens was then carefully dissected (it leads from the testicle proper to the seminal vescicle), with special care not to damage the tiny blood vessels that accompany it and supply the testes. The vas deferens was then ligated with silk sutures and finally divided.

The site of the ligation was at first the point where the vas leaves the testicle. During later operations the position where the tiny sperm-carrying canals leave the testicle to collect in the epididymis was the ligature site. This second and favoured technique became known as the Steinach II operation in subsequent literature. After operation the skin was closed with sutures and the wound powdered with an antiseptic substance. The rat was then wrapped in cotton wool to recover from the operation. This generally took about an hour, after which the senile rat moved about his cage and started to feed. After a few days the sutures were removed and the animal appeared to have recovered from its ordeal.

In about three to four weeks there was a striking change in the animal's behaviour. Rats that had previously shown signs of senility rapidly became apparently younger. Their coats improved and they gradually became more active. Performance of a standardized strength test improved and appetite increased. The animals became heavier, subcutaneous fat and muscular tissue being responsible for this change. To use Steinach's own words, "his bearing is youthful and courageous, his ears are held upright and alert, and his eyes are wide open, clear and lively as of old and mirroring inquisitiveness for everything that takes place around him". More significantly to our subject, "on being brought in contact with females he will give convincing proof of his awakened virility".[87]

When these animals were sacrificed it was found that a tremendous proliferation of tissue had taken place in the seminal vesicles. Steinach was able to demonstrate also that this proliferation and rejuvenation occurred just as well if only one vas deferens was divided at operation. In these cases the rejuvenated rats were not sterile and mated successfully, producing normal offspring. Although the numbers of animals used in the experiments were not large by modern standards, Steinach successfully rejuvenated a series of over fifty senile animals.

Steinach argued that his operation was merely an artificial stimulation of a normal physiological process. He believed in what he called the "struggle of the parts". By tying the normal duct of the external secretion of the testes the cells that produced the spermatozoa degenerated and the interstitial tissue of the testes proliferated. This was followed by greater output of the sex hormone produced by this tissue.

Gradually Steinach elaborated his researches. He found that a stage could be reached at which rats were too old to be rejuvenated. Also that after the Steinach II operation the blood supply to the brain appeared to be increased. Further studies in conjunction with Dr. E. Lost of Vienna proved transient rejuvenation possible by means of diathermy experiments. Guinea pigs were used for these tests and even castrated animals responded to some extent. Steinach thought this was due to an increase in oxygen and hormone transportation brought about by hyperaemia of the tissues.

Further studies of old rats, rejuvenated by vasoligation, showed that at least partial histological rejuvenation of ageing tissues, both in body muscles and cardiac musculature, could be demonstrated, and that eye lens and corneal opacities cleared. Experiments with dogs apparently nearly blind with senile cataract showed them able to get their bearings, see objects and avoid obstructions a few weeks after the Steinach II operation.

The year 1921 saw Steinach very much involved with the veterinary profession in Europe, Russia and North and South America. Broadly speaking, it seemed that vasectomy had a similar effect on senile dogs as he had demonstrated with rats and by now men of science were beginning to look towards Steinach quite seriously as the father of a new surgical speciality—Rejuvenation.

Steinach, of course, had no experience of human surgery. He had, however, a young Viennese urological surgeon, Robert Lichtenstern, working in his laboratory as far back as 1918, who was enthusiastic enough about Steinach's work on experimental animals to be persuaded to carry out the first Steinach I operation on man for the purposes of rejuvenation. Of course the operation of vasectomy (division of the vas deferens) had been performed before and was popular as early as 1890 in Sweden as a treatment for enlarged prostate. But on 1st November, 1918, Lichtenstern's first patient submitted to operation for quite different reasons.

Unfortunately Steinach's clinical notes on this man, Anton W., a coachman of forty-three, do not make it quite sure that he was suffering from anything much more than endogenous depression. He complained of being extremely exhausted and miserable, had difficulty in breathing, poor appetite and loss of weight. Physical examination showed wasted musculature, a dull, dry skin, receding hair, scanty beard and bronchitis. He had a normal cardiovascular system.

After operation there was no appreciable change for two or three months, but then quite suddenly improvement took place. Although living was difficult in Vienna at this time as a result of the first world war and meat was virtually absent from the diet, the patient regained his strength and appetite. His skin texture improved and he became much more hirsute. A year later he was thirty-five pounds heavier than when he was operated upon. Six months later still, it was noted that the patient now possessed "a smooth, unwrinkled face. His smart and upright bearing gives the impression of a youthful man at the height of his vitality".

Obviously the publication of this case and others that followed of an essentially similar nature greatly excited surgeons with an experimental turn of mind, and during the 1920s literally hundreds of men were operated upon with favourable results, notably by Lichtenstern and Peter Schmidt in Germany, H. Benjamin in America and Norman Haire and Kenneth Walker in London. Rejuvenation by surgery boomed to a fantastic degree and case history after case history was published in the medical, paramedical and lay press.

Considering the *genre* of surgical practice of the times, many of the accounts published make impressive reading even today. Dr. Peter Schmidt of Berlin was a clever operator in his day and possessed a scientific outlook. In his main writings on the subject [86] he advised that pre-operatively patients should be photographed, their temperature and coloration of the ears and extremities should be carefully noted together with their body weight. Muscular strength should be measured on a dynamometer, also blood pressure and pulse rate. The urine should be examined and a careful general physical examination carried out. Finally a blood count and Wasserman reaction should be recorded together with details of any history of gonorrhea. The question of relative sexual potency completed the pre-operative clinical history.

After operation Schmidt counted increased elasticity and colour of skin, changes in hair growth, weight gain, increase in physical strength, decrease in blood pressure, improvement in vasomotor function, improvement in eyesight, increase in appetite, improvement in arteriosclerotic symptoms and increase or reappearance of libido as signs of rejuvenation, together with psychic changes which can be summarized as increase in mental facility, energy and *joie de vivre*.

Schmidt claimed that in half the cases he operated upon there was complete rejuvenation after four to six months, and that the effects lasted several years. In other cases there was partial success. Other authors reported similar results. Norman Haire and Kenneth M. Walker produced broadly similar results. Haire summarized his first hundred Steinach operations in these words. "A few patients do not show any improvement, physical, mental or sexual, though I have never seen a patient who was adversely affected by it. The great majority show physical and mental improvement, and most experience improvement in the sexual sphere as well." Haire wrote convincingly about various rejuvenation techniques, and his opinions are summarized in his book.[89]

In 1932 Dr. Harry Benjamin of New York summed up his experience of the Steinach therapy over the previous ten years.[93] He admitted that his initial attitude towards the Steinach operation was more than sceptical, and that over the ten years in question his enthusiasm waxed and waned. Nevertheless he had come to the conclusion that Steinach's operation was of undoubted value. Analysing his results based on operations on over

500 men, he judged his success rate to be about 75 per cent. These positive results lasted, according to the patient's age, from one and a half to six years. A successful case, according to Benjamin, displayed subjective and objective signs of improved endocrine function after operation. The most common subjective improvements were with reference to exhaustion, insomnia, inability to concentrate, general irritability and lack of appetite. As far as objective findings, there was a lowering of blood pressure, improved hair growth, improved skin texture and improved eyesight and hearing. In 1932 Benjamin's considered opinion was that "endocrine reactivation methods, if applied properly and estimated conservatively, can be a blessing to many".[94]

Gradually, however, counterblasts against Steinach gained in volume and dismal reports of failures started to creep into the medical journals. Often these were refuted by the successful operators on the grounds that imperfect surgical techniques were complicating the picture. Steinach only recommended that the seminal ducts should be tied, the vascular and nervous tissues all being left intact, and the clear implication was that the critics were not following this method efficiently.

At a meeting of prominent Austrian surgeons and physiologists on 21st January, 1928, Dr. Schoenbauer of the Eilenberg Clinic claimed that he had only come across one patient who had derived benefit from vasoligation, and suggested that autosuggestion had played a part in all successful rejuvenation operations. Steinach enthusiasts, however, were not slow to point out counter-arguments.

Clayton E. Wheeler, another supporter of Steinach in the US asked, "what sort of auto-suggestion was employed by those senile octogenarian rats dying on their feet, not able to stand on their hind feet and reach up for food suspended in their cage, but who after vasectomy by Steinach became active, kept themselves clean, fed voraciously, fought the younger males introduced into their cage for possession of the female, copulated and brought forth healthy rat broods; all at a time when they should, according to rat chronology, have been long dead and in the incinerator?".[95] Dr. Wheeler also quoted "hundreds of men" who had been vasectomized for the purpose of sterilization in the US because they were "degenerate, criminal or insane" and who had only been told that their procreative ability might be abolished and yet suddenly found themselves startlingly rejuvenated. Their digestion improved, their metabolic rate was raised, their hair quality and quantity was also improved and "impotence, often of years standing, was relieved and virility once more restored".

But on the whole an impression is left that surgeons eventually became completely disenchanted with Steinach's operation. Kenneth Macfarlane Walker, the British surgeon and author, gives the lie to this impression. Writing recently of his own experiences,[96] he allowed that the results of the operations done on thousands of men in the previous twenty years were found to be disappointing and inferior to those previously obtained by Steinach in his animal experiments. He thought, however, that it was not easy to assess human results on this score, for many patients felt themselves greatly benefited by the operation, although objective evidence was not always so convincing. Looking back on his own records Walker opined that a third of his patients "were satisfied with what they believed themselves to have gained . . . a third considered that there had been some slight improvement in their condition: in the remaining third the results were entirely negative".

Another more likely reason for a declining interest in the twenties in Steinach's work was the appearance of a new star in the firmament of rejuvenation ideology, that of Serge Voronoff. Dapper, effervescent Voronoff, taking to himself an extremely pretty young wife in 1931 when he was already sixty-five, was every inch the classical rejuvenationist. Believed to be Russian, Voronoff's early life is hedged in obscurity. In all probability he emigrated to France in 1892 to practise surgery and pathology. Apparently his early days of surgical practice in France were unrewarding, for the first firm mention of him prior to 1914 was as physician surgeon to Abbas II Khedive of Egypt.

While working in Egypt Voronoff had the opportunity to observe at first hand the characteristics of the eunuchs in local harems, and it is said that these observations, curiously, fired in him an undying interest in the physiology of sex. During the war years the life of a young surgeon took a more practical turn and Voronoff forged for himself a career of some distinction in military hospital work. Eventually he was appointed director of the laboratory of experimental surgery at the Collège de France.

In the early days at the Collège Voronoff toyed with the idea of testicular transplantation for cases in which, due to age or "testicular exhaustion or deficiency due to congenital causes, some local change such as orchitis or sclerosis" had taken place.[87] Unfortunately for his researches adequate supplies of human tissue were not forthcoming. French law forbade the use of cadaveric material obtained as a result of accidents, and although Voronoff explored the possibility of obtaining tissues from criminals condemned to death, this was finally abandoned. These fundamental setbacks are said to have led Voronoff along another line—that of using anthropoid apes as donors of testicular tissue. In 1920, on 13th June, Voronoff carried out his first ape-to-man testicular transplant, and in the next two years 162 similar operations were conducted. Voronoff's operations could hardly he expected to go unnoticed in Paris at this time and the newspapers reacted in a strictly predictable way, enthusing wildly over his apparent success. So much so that the new Professor Voronoff was thought by his professional colleagues not to be a proper person to read a paper at the French Academy of Medicine on the occasion of the thirty-first Congress of French Surgeons.

Some three months after the publication of his first successful operation Voronoff, never a bashful man and furious at being muzzled at the recent Congress, counteracted by giving a press conference at which he presented tripartate evidence in the shape of an old man, a billy goat and a ram, all apparently rejuvenated by testicular transplants from apes. Naturally enough this produced a sensation and "thousands of articles were published about him, religious sects and antivivisectionists attacked him, though for different reasons, cartoons depicted grandfathers swinging from chandeliers, the monkey gland fever broke the thermometer".[33]

The fame of "monkey gland" rejuvenation, of course, soon

rebounded on Voronoff, and men of science, albeit unconsciously, turned aside from him and he gradually became an object of ridicule. If, however, Voronoff's writings are examined in a dispassionate light, although as a scientist he was clearly no Steinach, his logic, surgical techniques and results need more serious consideration than they have received. Although Voronoff is primarily remembered as rejuvenationist in his early work, he explored many other aspects of gland transplantation therapy.

His indications of testicular transplantation included congenital or accidental loss of the testes, infantilism of the sexual organs, delayed puberty, arteriosclerosis, schizophrenia and neurotic illness, as well as senility whether physiological or premature.

Voronoff's operating technique is fully documented. The donor monkey was anaesthetized with chloroform, its skin shaved and sterilized. The patient was anaesthetized, simultaneously either by local or general methods. Two surgeons worked together, one opening the monkey's scrotum and removing the testicle, together with its covering, the tunica vaginalis. The other operator then cut down through the patient's scrotum. While the monkey's testicle was being removed from its tunica, and being sliced into six pieces longitudinally, the other surgeon carefully stitched the grafts either to the patient's tunica vaginalis on its outer surface (three on to each testicle), or if a sufficiently large sac surrounded the testicle the transplant was stitched on to the inside of this membrane. The incision in the tunica was then closed. Voronoff believed that each graft should be sutured with silk quite separately to get the best implantation results. Usually his patients rested for a few days after operation, although this was not insisted upon.

Voronoff was careful not to claim that all his cases were successful or that sexual rejuvenation always occurred. Quite often too he admitted that the effects of glandular implantations lasted only a relatively short time, a period on the average of eighteen months to three years.

By 1928 the medical profession in Europe, although hesitating to accept Voronoff's treatments as true rejuvenation, had moved to the position of publicly acknowledging that they had some therapeutic effect. A conference of a thousand leading surgeons in Austria met in January 1928 and agreed that although "rejuvenation" as such was a misnomer, "the gland transplantation operation devised by Dr. Serge Voronoff afforded transient regeneration".[97]

One of Voronoff's prize cases of rejuvenation was not a man but an old ram that had been kept alive and healthy far beyond its normal life span by means of gland grafting from a human:

> A ram, twelve to fourteen years old corresponding to about eighty years in man, which could hardly totter, received an implant of testicle fragment from a young man. Two months after the graft had been effected, the animal was completely transformed. His urinal incontinence had disappeared so had tremblings of the legs, and he was no longer looking afraid. His bodily carriage had become magnificent, and he behaved in a lively and aggressive manner. The old ram had taken on the appearance of remarkable youth and vigour. He was isolated in a small stable with a young ewe lamb, which afforded the opportunity for observing not only the reawakening of the sex instincts which he had lost years ago, but also the following more tangible results. The ewe lamb covered by him in September . . . dropped a vigorous lamb in February.[98]

Naturally enough the veterinary profession and animal breeders were extremely interested in such work. Voronoff's experiments suddenly received national patronage and the French government voted a law prohibiting the hunting of chimpanzees, the animals becoming protected and reserved for Voronoff's experiments. This move was apparently not successful in providing all the material needed and eventually the British and Belgian governments gave Voronoff's agents permission to capture animals in their territories in Africa.

Strangely it was from the world of veterinary science that the first powerful blow fell that raised serious doubts, not only about Voronoff the rejuvenator but of Voronoff the scientist. A delegation made up of a physiologist, a geneticist, a dietician and a veterinary surgeon was sent by the British Ministry of Agriculture to Algiers to inquire into Voronoff's cattle-breeding improvement schemes. Once at work they pursued their studies ruthlessly. Their conclusions spelt scientific disaster as far as British and American opinion was concerned.

A bull discarded as useless at the age of seventeen was said to have sired nine calves in two years after the Voronoff operation. The delegation raised the objection that there was doubt in the paternity of the calves in question and asked the pointed question as to why, when a bull was normally slaughtered at the age of twelve in Algiers, this particular animal had been kept alive another five years, long past its normal breeding age.

Flocks of sheep were then inspected as to the quality and quantity of wool they produced after rejuvenation. They inquired as to the details of numbers of animals used and their pedigrees, but found satisfactory information "not forthcoming". Such animals as were used in the experiments were not confined under proper experimental conditions and nutritional factors were ignored.

All in all, the British delegation were not impressed. In summing up their visit they were cagey but unenthusiastic. Claims to rejuvenate the aged and decrepit, they argued, might be justified. But the evidence they had examined was not based on critical experimentation, and as far as cattle-rearing and livestock improvement were concerned they could find no economic advantages in Voronoff's methods.[99]

The nineteen-twenties and thirties were in many ways the hey-day of new ideas on the subject of sexual and general rejuvenation. A persual of the medical journals of the world at this time gives ample support to this statement, for every few months fresh scientific papers were being published on the subject. In many cases they were mere extensions of previously tried methods that owed intellectual allegiance to the master minds of Steinach and Brown-Séquard.

Typical of many of these was "Doppler's method", named after Dr. Karl Doppler of Vienna. Originally hailed by the *New York Times* with the acclamation that "no operation or transplantation is necessary. . . . 200 cases successfully treated in two years",[100] enthusiasts on seeing Dr. Doppler were doubtless rather disappointed to find that an operation, albeit a minor one, *was* necessary. An incision was made in the inguinal region, and the arterial supply to the testes was dissected out and brushed with a 7 per cent solution of phenol. This procedure was carried out with a view to paralysing the sympathetic nerves round the arterial wall and causing the artery to dilate, thus theoretically improving the blood supply to the testes.

The Doppler method certainly seemed to work, if one can judge by the published results. Apparently there was not only sexual rejuvenation but also very marked psychological improvement. Senile deafness disappeared, hair began to thicken or become darker. Patients became more energetic and youthful. Needless to say, the Doppler technique had its own retinue of protagonists on a world-wide basis for several years and scientific papers were published on the subject in medical journals as late as the year 1939.

Naturally enough some methods that seemed particularly effective in the 1920s soon dropped from favour when further intrinsic scientific knowledge eventually adjudged them to be potentially damaging and possibly lethal. Steinach himself had carried out experiments in which the sex glands were irradiated with X-rays. Working with immature female guinea pigs he carefully screened off the upper body and the animal below the pelvis with lead and then subjected the abdomen to X-ray irradiation. Using untreated identical animals as controls Steinach proved conclusively that the secondary sexual characteristics of the females developed much quicker in the irradiated animals. On examination of the irradiated ovaries there was a striking absence of grafian follicles but a greater proliferation of the hormone producing interstitial tissue.

Other experiments showed that similar effects on males occurred and that sterilization was easy by the judicious use of X-ray in animals; secondary sexual characteristics becoming more florid and developing with some precociousness. Eventually Krisen and Lenk of Vienna applied similar treatments to elderly men who had been virtually impotent for years. As might be expected these patients showed an increasing deficiency in their sperm count as treatment progressed. On the other hand the "Steinach effect" was produced. Their vigour and potency increased considerably. Dr. H. Benjamin in the US was for some

time a staunch supporter of the rejuvenation of women by radio-
therapy, and fearlessly published his successes and failures. The
cases reported by Norman Haire [89] show that the women reacted
extremely well to the therapy and both looked and felt very much
younger.

Today, of course, the use of X-ray therapy to the gonads is
strictly confined to the treatment of certain aspects of malignant
disease. The risks of inducing cancerous lesions by the indis-
criminate use of X-rays is judged to be too great for any non-
essential use to be justified.

The fertile brain of Steinach also brought into being another
rejuvenation vogue of the late 1920s, rejuvenation by diathermy.
As previously mentioned, Steinach found that mature castrates
could maintain virtual sexual normality provided they were given
daily abdominal diathermy treatment. Dr. Peter Schmidt applied
similar therapy to women, giving ovarian diathermy five times
weekly over a period of from four to six weeks. The results of
this rather protracted therapy appears to have been rather disappointing.

An extension of Brown-Séquard's work was made in the late
1920s by several American surgeons, notably L. L. Stanley of
California. Stanley had begun his interest in the subject by practising a Voronoff technique but using human testicles taken from
recently executed convicts at San Quentin Penitentiary. Later he
substituted rams' testicles for human organs and found these to
be just as effective. He favoured an abdominal site for implantation, rather than Voronoff's scrotal one and came to the conclusion that testicular material used in this way had a stimulating
and invigorating effect upon the recipient sexually as well as
mentally and physically.

Later he extended his researches into a field subsequently explored more thoroughly by Niehans (see chapter 7). Using a
suspension of chopped-up fragments of rams' and goats' testes,
he injected it subcutaneously into volunteer patients at the California State Prison. The lumps of foreign protein could be felt
as bean-like nodules under the skin for some months. The main
interest in the procedure lies in the relatively large number of

patients involved, some 656 in all, and the large number of those who benefited. Although such experimentation must have had very heavy psychological overtones, the published reports show that subjectively, at any rate, the convicts were vastly improved by the treatment.[101]

Subsequently Professor Karenchevsky at the Lister Institute in London prepared extracts of bulls' testes for a similar series of tests carried out at St. Mary Abbots hospital in conjunction with the National Institute of Industrial Psychology. From the point of view of rejuvenation, however, the results were entirely negative.

Elsewhere in the world, however, Stanley-type rejuvenation boomed. Dr. Albert Schneider, in an interesting review of the whole of rejuvenation, written in 1928,[102] estimated that at that time some 50,000 Stanley operations had been carried out in the US and in all probability many more than that number in Europe "with quite uniformly good results and without ill effects".

Gradually, with the passing of the 1930s, interest in rejuvenation by means of sex glands or their extracts waned. Fewer and fewer papers on the subject were published, and one gets the impression that the experimental minds that had previously devoted themselves to the subject shone their inquisitive light elsewhere. Here and there, however, there were echoes of the past. In 1947 K. V. Matthew of the Karura Hospital in Madras published his own results on vasectomy carried out over the years from 1933 to 1946. The series was not large (106 cases were described), but only nine were reported as having had no effect. Two-thirds of his cases reported themselves cured of impotence and there were the usual mentions of hair colour being restored. An amusing but apparently sincere personal report quoted can hardly have put the matter more picturesquely: "I have the least hesitation in saying that the wonderful operation you performed on me at Alleppy has had glorious results. In short, it is this operation that has thrown open the gates of heaven to me".[103]

There seems little doubt that the second world war, with its redirection of so many national interests, finally extinguished organized scientific research on the sex glands and their relation-

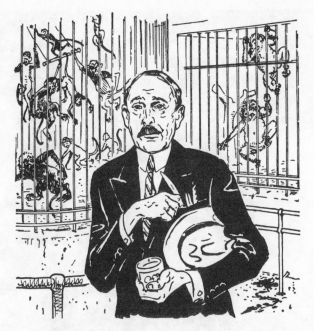

Voronoff with some of his famous monkeys.
Inscribed "Beware Voronoff's coming!"

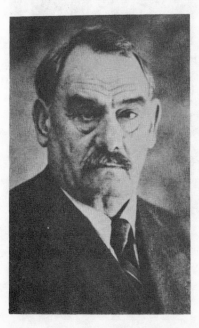 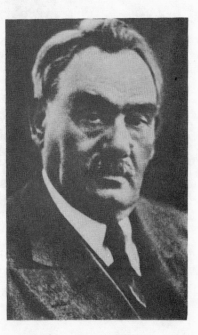

Voronoff's elder brother before and after rejuvenation

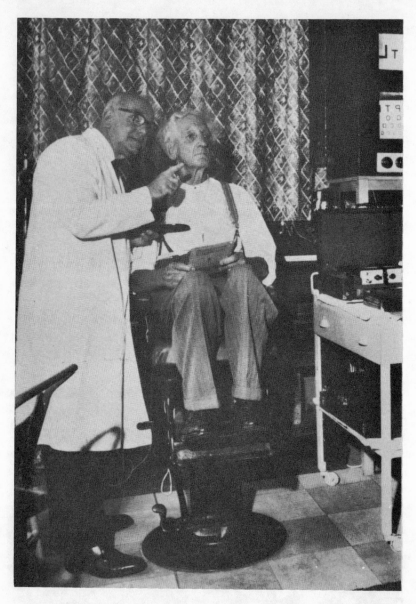

Dr. John Maddison engaged in testing an elderly patient's visual acuity at the experimental clinic for preventive medicine for older people at Teddington, Middlesex

ship to rejuvenation. The dawn of the antibiotic age was also coming and the tremendous change it made in surgical practice must have affected the history of rejuvenation. Many new fields of surgical practice were opened up and surgeons' enthusiasm for the extension of other aspects of their work in all probability redirected many energies. In some ways it would seem that a candle was snuffed out prematurely on this score, although many thinking medical men earnestly believed there to be a big future for the subject for several decades. Albert Schneider, M.S., PH.D., M.D., previously quoted,[104] felt that too great a tribute could not be paid to the research of Steinach, Voronoff, Lydston, Thorek, Kammener, Stanley and Benjamin for their courage in continuing efforts in a new field of human endeavour despite the opposition of their colleagues and the alternating ridicule and clamorous support of the popular press.

He also felt that the destruction of the ancient libraries of Africa, Arabia, China and Greece had robbed medicine of much of potential value to the rejuvenationist and implored scholars to study the remaining sources of ancient medical lore available in Indian, Chinese and Persian writings. Clayton E. Wheeler of Los Angeles, California, wrote in similar vein to the *Medical Journal and Record* in 1928, when he compared the intolerant attitude towards the work of the experimental and practising rejuvenationist to that displayed towards anaesthetists in the 1840s and to the work of Lister and Pasteur when it was first published: "We are sneering and mocking at the thing that might make us complete men and women and give us from two to ten, or even fifteen years more of healthy happy existence on this plane of experience".

Although in London, parts of the US and in Europe it is still possible to find medical men of repute and enthusiasm who are actively involved in the practice of rejuvenation through methods analogous to those we have examined in this chapter, professional enthusiasm today is at a minimum. The stigma of a reputable doctor using "monkey gland" therapy is apparently a hard one to surmount.

10

Bee Nonsense and other Curiosities

It is often difficult to separate quack from paramedical or unorthodox medicine. Some writers see almost an open warfare between the "professionals" in any field, with their vested interest in tradition and a monopoly of learning and the innovators who question oracular authority.[105] Brian Inglis takes the argument a little further and sees what amounts to virtual blackleg treatment handed out by the hierarchy of the medical profession to "doctors who are attracted to unorthodox ideas", and claims that this deters the profession from "enriching itself by absorbing fresh ideas from unorthodoxy" because of possible fear and ridicule.[106]

There is no doubt, of course, that ideas in the history of rejuvenation have suffered because of the fear of professional ridicule. But there is little real evidence that such criticism has very much effect on the fringe medicine of rejuvenation, and many curious ideas still hold sway.

One of the most interesting of these curiosities that had a short-lived but reasonably successful life was Royal Jelly. From the strictly scientific point of view there is nothing very exciting about Royal Jelly, and it is bound up intimately with the social life of bees. The hive bee (*Apis mellifera*) has a more intricate existence than other bees. Differences between queens, drones and workers are pronounced. Part of the social activity of the young workers is to secrete from glands under the abdomen a wax for comb building. This they mould into the cells of the honey-comb which are shaped in one of these ways: cells to house future workers are small, numerous and regular; the compartments that will house drones are larger and less stereotyped; while those for the future queen are in the form of irregular sacs. The queen bee lays an egg in each brood cell, and when the young larvae hatch out they have three possible fates: if the eggs are unfertilized they develop into drones; if the eggs are fertilized they may either become queens or worker bees, and diet seems to control exactly what happens in these cases.

All larvae are fed first of all on a product of the salivary glands of worker bees, known as royal jelly. Those who are destined to become queen bees remain on this diet until they are adult. Other bees, workers or drones, are subsequently fed on a pollen and honey mixture.

The magazine *Family Doctor*, published by the British Medical Association, enjoyed a unique position in medical journalism. Its editorial policy revolved around a few unarguable considerations, the first of which was "Is it medically correct?" It also faced up to real problems, avoided medical jargon and scientific mumbo jumbo. Most important, it waged a constant protective war in favour of the patient, a war which is sometimes directed against paramedical adventurers whose claims seemed, on careful con-sideration, to be curious and misleading.

In February 1958 Dr. Harvey Flack, medical historian and founder editor of *Family Doctor* magazine, took the question of royal jelly and its commercialization as "Apiserum" as the sub-ject for his monthly editor's letter. Readers had written to the magazine asking for a medical opinion on "Apiserum", which was supposed to be royal jelly that can retard old age. Dr. Flack in his wisdom explained that royal jelly had been carefully studied and that it contained high proportions of the vitamins of the B group, notably pantothenic acid and biotin, but sensibly assured his readers that no ordinary diet could be envisaged that lacked adequate amounts of these substances.

Nevertheless he accepted the fact that royal jelly could possibly contain an unidentified substance, capable of transforming a larva into a queen bee, and that this supposed substance might be good for us to eat. Going on to point out quite quietly and scientifically that different sized animals needed different daily quantities of things like vitamins, roughly in proportion to their size, he made a razor-sharp observation. Presuming, for the sake of argument, that the average man weighed about the same as a million bee larvae, he continued, "I guess that I need to eat the amount of royal jelly supplied to at least fifty thousand larvae each day to have any effect on me, always assuming, of course, that this un-identified, unknown, unproved magic does exist in royal jelly". He went on to state that this would mean "thousands of people working with thousands of beehives . . . extracting the royal jelly out of the glands of the nursing bees. . . . I should think they would have their work cut out to get enough to have any effect on one solitary person". Another characteristic of *Family Doctor* maga-zine was a distinct tendency to consult the expert whenever an opinion seemed in any way in doubt, and in this case a prominent professor of nutrition from London University opined "I just don't believe in it. First, I don't really believe that there is any miraculous substance in royal jelly which will do for me what good, straight fish and chips can't do. And second, if there were such a stuff, I don't believe there is enough in your five guineas' worth of Apiserum to make the slightest difference to me, even if I consumed it all in one day." Dr. Harvey Flack concluded that "bee nonsense" was the right sort of reply to give to anyone who tried to sell you royal jelly at "five guineas a go". Nevertheless thousands of people parted with their guineas and put their faith in the bees.

Honey as a rejuvenating substance, either "neat" or as a "Honegar" (equal parts of apple cider, vinegar and pure honey), received a tremendous boost as a result of a book written by a doctor from Vermont, US,[107] who had practised in the "Green Mountain State" for over fifty years. Impressed by the fact that Vermonters were extremely long-lived, having the second largest proportion of inhabitants over the age of sixty-five in the US, he set about trying to find the reason for this and found it to his own satisfaction in folk medicine.

One of his pet theories was that honey, being a mixture of

levulose and dextrose, had a "selective" action on blood sugar that
was protective and health-giving. Although the rationale behind
his reasoning remains scientifically obscure his readers obviously
believed in its therapeutic effect and thousand of citizens of the
US alone were soon either drinking Honegar or "mixing their
own" at home. ("Two teaspoons of honey and two teaspoons of
apple cider vinegar taken in a glass of water one or more times
a day. The blend tastes like a glass of apple cider. The vinegar
brings across from the apple its mineral content, the honey brings
across the minerals in the nectar of flowers.") [107]

Later, Dr. Jarvis found other therapeutic uses for honey. It
killed typhoid and dysentery germs, it was useful for infant feeding, it cured bedwetting, as well as insomnia. "Muscle cramps"
eased off before its powerful action, it cured coughs or could be
used as a burn dressing. Athletes were recommended to train on
it and if you chewed a honeycomb it banished catarrh, hay fever
and sinusitis. This was, naturally enough, rather too wide a spectrum of therapeutic beneficence to impress anyone with a
scientific turn of mind.

Far removed from honey chemically, but close to it in folksy
character, is the rejuvenation idea of Marguerite Maury. Madame
Maury, little known in Britain or the US, has a considerable
following in Europe, although few would agree with a statement
made by her English publishers that "her list of grateful clients
and successful cures encompasses the globe". Her method, to
quote her own words, is "rejuvenation through essential Oils—
a Modern Alchemy". The exact techniques she uses are a trifle
obscure, but somehow she believes that "in the odiferous molecule
modern biology has recognized the most subtle form of living
material, the dynamic, stimulating and palliative spirit of Nature's
formidable drive".

Her basic ideas on the rejuvenation are sensible enough, for she
confesses that she feels that victory over old age can be gained
only if we "contemplate and reflect on its nature from all sides".
Madame Maury has obviously read pretty widely the medical
and paramedical literature of rejuvenation, but does not always
seem to have used her knowledge to its best scientific purpose.

Fundamental to her theories is a conception of the "locunary liquid" which forms "part of the mass circulating in the body, on a par with the blood, the lymph and . . . the humours". This locunary liquid would seem to merely be another name for the plasma, for it circulates through the "extra-cellular space" of the body and occupies an area that she has calculated to represent 27.5 per cent of the volume of the body. Upon the quality of the locunary liquid, Madame Maury assumes, depends the "life of the cell, its rhythm and its pulsation". When the fluid becomes depleted or deranged, old age advances.

This is not the only rather strange physiological theory of the high priestess of aromatherapy. She also has great difficulty in separating the changes brought about in the body by pathological processes from those that are more conventionally looked upon as being due to senility. For example, children who contract arthritis she looks upon as being the "young old". Sexual debility or lack of libido to the extent of impotence she puts down to precocious sexuality, "just as a fruit plucked from the tree before it is ripe decays more swiftly, a young human being unprepared and brought into brutal contact with reality fades rapidly".

Madame Maury alleges that the source material of her theories are the "three thousand year old Ayurvedas . . . of Tibetan Medicine". The essences used she considers to be the vegetable hormones that are present in the "plasma" of various plants. These perfumes, as we might reasonably judge them to be, "regulate the activity of the capillaries" when applied to the skin, and "make the flesh more succulent". But another greater effect is supposedly brought about due to the fragrance of the essence that causes powers of perception to clear, and emotional troubles to disappear. The conscious mind is alerted and strength and youth are preserved.

Odoriferous matter brings the blood its indispensable and sovereign element. Its precious matter seeps into the biological liquids which carry it along and convey it throughout the whole body. Then a true regeneration occurs. The building of tissue is best observed when wounds are treated with this substance. There will be no scar, and burns will leave no trace.[108]

Naturally enough the author has her own particular methods and various different "odoriferous substances" are applied to the skin. She makes a great point in formulating an individual prescription for each patient (the I.P.), thus maintaining personal contact with her flock and making mass commercialization impossible.

Madame Maury in the best tradition of rejuvenation quotes from her case histories. Unfortunately the cases given are quite inadequate as far as any medical judgement is concerned. One of her prize cases quoted was a woman of fifty-five, an early age for rejuvenation by anyone's yardstick, who was a "small, frail, faded woman with a grey skin and grey hair. . . . Her character had more or less died. She took no pleasure in anything and lapsed into this *grisaille* despite quite a pleasant material situation." Treatment consisted of an I.P. of *elemi*, *galbanum*, violet leaves and lemon grass. The first two ingredients are, incidentally, used by Egyptian embalmers for impregnating mummy bandages. After two months' treatment the patient was "truly rejuvenated. Her complexion was pink, her gait and behaviour youthful, she slept better, was gay and had even fallen in love."

The ideas held on rejuvenation by an intelligent cosmetologist —who prefaces her book with a testimonial from the Marchioness of Reading—and an emeritus director of the Kiev Institute of Experimental Biology and Pathology—who was at one time called upon to rejuvenate Joseph Stalin—would seem to have little in common. Both, however, believe that the secret of ageing lies in the body fluids. The former believed fundamentally that this could be altered by applying perfumes to the skin. The latter felt that, as the cells in the body of the reticulo-endothelial system seem to remain constantly fully functional and therefore youthful, a serum that would stimulate the cells of this system would *ipso facto* through the body fluids retard degeneration and prevent ageing.

Dr. Alexander Bogomolets was born in 1881 and his early days read like a tale from Dostoevsky or Tolstoy. His mother was a young medical student accused by the Tsarist regime of revolutionary activity, who after being imprisoned at the Lubianovka prison in Kiev was sentenced to live in exile in Siberia. Young Bogomolets was brought up by his grandfather, a retired Army officer who had served under Nicholas I, and was eventually sent to the University of Odessa to study medicine. Graduating with high honours at the age of twenty-five, he was appointed to the department of general pathology at Odessa, where he worked for five years before leaving to take up a professorship of pathology at Saratov.

Bogomolets survived the onslaught of the first world war, and the subsequent revolution, as a consulting epidemiologist on the South West front, and when things had settled down was appointed to the second Moscow University as Professor of Pathology. His early interests were in the field of endocrinology and blood transfusion, and he was forty-nine before he devoted himself to the study of rejuvenation as the founder and director of the famous Kiev Institute, Here, aided by a large staff, Bogomolets first of all studied cellular biology and then turned his attention to tissue ageing.

His general ideas on rejuvenation were quite orthodox. He subscribed to the theory that as far as the animal world was concerned the life span is usually five to six times the period it takes a species to reach maturity, and that mankind therefore should live to 125 or 150 years. Old age was defined as the loss of the ability of the organism to regenerate, and he placed this as a basic failure of the cells of what he called the "physiological system of the connective tissue".

Translators in the Western world suggest that these cells may be the fixed histiocytes found in the connective tissue, the spleen, lymphatic glands, bone marrow, the cells of the endothelial structures in the spleen, liver and endocrine glands, the microglia of the nervous system, and the wandering histocytes in the tissue spaces of the body. Included as well in this general category are the fibroblasts of the connective tissue. Here at once we seem to be struggling with nomenclature and terminology, and this is unfortunate because Bogomolets' main contribution to the history of rejuvenation involves a "serum" made from cells of what he calls the "physiologic system of connective tissue" and injecting it into the old and ageing, and so it is particularly important to define these cells accurately.

Curiously enough Bogomolets' theory is an extension of some late work of Metchnikoff (*see* chapter 6), under whose influence he came in his early medical career. Metchnikoff's dictum that the fight against old age should be directed towards strengthening the more vulnerable elements of the body and weakening the "aggressiveness of the phagocytes" led on to a search for ways of strengthening organs in rather the same way as the organism as a whole can be strengthened against specific infections, that is, by the production of antibodies.

The general theory appears to be as follows. If, for instance, the liver or the testes would be "strengthened", then these cells are injected into an animal of another species. This obviously produces antibodies in the experimental animal, and if the process is repeated several times, these are found, eventually, in the blood of the animal. Small doses of this experimental serum were then reinjected into the person whose organs were to be stimulated, and it was felt that this gave a specific regenerative response.

Bogomolets started experiments along these lines, not as a rejuvenation technique but in an attempt to intensify the secretion of the adrenal glands. By elaborating an antiserum in the way previously described he produced what he called a specific cytotoxic serum from the adrenal glands. Now, believing, as he did, that the "cells of physiologic system of connecting tissue" not only were the basic mechanism by which the organism resisted infection but also were potentially responsible for combating the ravages of old age, it was logical to produce a specific cytotoxic serum made from those cells.

The exact method of production of this specific cytotoxic serum or ACS does not appear in translations of Bogomolets' work.[109] Nevertheless precise instructions were published in the 1940s for its clinical use. The cells from which it was made have, of course, a wide range of function, and are particularly active in all healing processes, infections and even malignant disease. The serum was therefore widely used in the treatment of fractures, in scarlet fever, typhus, tularemia, brucellosis, post-puerperal infections, acute rheumatism, syphilis and malaria. Cancer was also thought to be restrained if not cured by ACS, and, of course, ageing greatly retarded.

Bogomolets, however, remained reasonably level-headed amongst the enthusiasm for ACS, and stressed that together with measures to lengthen life it should always be remembered that the avoidance of factors that are known to shorten life are important.

In the West, scientists appear to have given ACS a fair clinical trial. They confirmed that it stimulated wound and fracture healing, but had no effect in biological life span.[110] In more recent years attempts have been made to revive the autoimmunological aspects of Bogomolets' thinking in the treatment of malignant disease, but results have not as yet been conclusive one way or the other.

Bogomolets' basic "keep fit" ideas and the avoidance of factors known to shorten life were sensible enough, and are reflected in much modern writing on this subject. This aspect of rejuvenation has, however, attracted its own particular quota of curiosities and none has been more flamboyant in his views than Dr. Arnold Lorand, who wrote his treatise on rejuvenation in an old monastery in Vienna, where he was given board and lodging by the kindly Capuchin fathers during the last two years of the first world war.

Something of the austere nature of his environment seems to have permeated the whole personality of Dr. Lorand when he came to put his ideas on paper.[111]

High on Dr. Lorand's list of evils to be avoided at all costs by those who wanted to live long was alcohol, which he felt quite convinced poisoned the liver and the thyroid gland. The lungs and the heart too were weakened, he felt by alcohol, and the blood vessels quickly developed arteriosclerosis under its influence. The kidneys developed "nephritis which markedly shortens life". All this would seem sinister enough, but it was only the beginning of Dr. Lorand's dogma. "What makes this butcher of humanity especially fatal," he thundered, "is that it not only destroys the drinker but also plunges his innocent descendants into misfortune, and even in many cases consigns them to an early grave." Dr. Lorand's definition of a "drinker" was pretty niggardly by modern social drinking levels, for anyone who drank more than two glasses of wine a day fell into this category.

The next great enemy of longevity, Dr. Lorand felt, was too much protein in the diet. This predisposed, he was sure, to arterio-sclerosis, diabetes, gout and kidney disease and, what was more significant, brought on other disasters, for it led "one into temp-tation to drink and smoke after a meal, for there is nothing that a full stomach desires so much as alcohol and tobacco".

Once launched on tobacco the good doctor was off on another sermon. Tobacco hardened the arteries and this curiously made smokers prone to syphilis. "I would like to mention the fact that there are people who, when asked, will admit that ten or twenty years before they had . . . a small scratch. . . ." which turned out to be syphilis. "It is a strange and tragic fact that as a rule it is these light cases that are in many circumstances the ones most to be feared . . . especially if strong tobacco has been used." Tobacco also he felt made people liable to apoplexy, constipation, sleep-lessness, dizziness, headache and failure of memory. Furthermore, it was, he felt, to be particularly poisonous to the "more frail structure and more delicate tissues" of women and young girls.

Fourth in line for bad marks as far as longevity was concerned was "sexual indiscretion". This led, in women, to "very serious disturbance of the sexual organs with consequences highly preju-dicial to their fertility and longevity". As far as men were con-cerned "sexual intoxication . . . love of Venus and Bacchus . . . the joys of rapture" are all very well at the time, Dr. Lorand agreed, but "many years later when the pains of body and mind torment him and when his innocent children are dying at an early age . . . he and all his companions in fate clench their fists towards heaven and wish they had neither loved nor drank".

But if sexual excess was a great danger, a greater one was "the avoidance of parenthood". The main reason for this, Lorand felt, was that a large family kept everyone very busy and "work is of Divine origin and a great protector of health". "Anticonceptional measures", he was sure, brought with them "serious disorders of the reproductive organs and of the nervous system" as well as arteriosclerosis and cancer. Dr. Lorand was a great devotee of cleanliness: "uncleanly persons may learn a lot from the bees", but warned his readers about the life-shortening dangers of ambition, "hundreds and thousands of American businessmen . . . are so consumed by it that they can never take time to enjoy a walk around the wonders of nature". He also advised against avarice—"greed and avarice shorten life"—not to mention anger —"it may bring on an attack of breast pang, the dreaded angina pectoris". Strangely too, and intent in going right through the seven deadly sins, Dr. Lorand listed vanity as a life-shortener: "very serious effects on the liver and bile circulation may be caused by tight lacing".

Although Dr. Lorand's ideas on the prolongation of life immediately brings to mind the innate query, "Is it worth it?", as far as he was concerned personally the answer was "Yes", for strangely he advocated the methods of Steinach and Voronoff. He also believed in the rejuvenating powers of thyroid extract, iodides, and ultraviolet light either in the form of sunlight or artificially from quartz lamps. Finally he was extremely enthusiastic about the rejuvenating properties of mud baths and radium baths, particularly for women.

Looking back on Lorand's work from the distance of forty or more years, it is incredible how wrong any one person can be when they ruthlessly ride a hobby horse. Alcohol, unless taken in pretty large quantities over a prolonged period, seems to have little effect on longevity. A high-protein diet is, contrary to his credo, a health scorer. "Sexual indiscretion" hardly seems to enter into the picture and contraception, as far as women are concerned, has resulted in their living longer. Anger expressed and acted out is probably less damaging to the psyche than anger suppressed, and it is doubtful if avarice or vanity are valid causes of an early demise.

Even when Dr. Lorand was right it was often for the wrong reasons. Tobacco kills mainly as a result of its action on the bronchial epithelium, although some would agree that it also is ultimately tied up with the development of arteriosclerosis and coronary thrombosis. Voronoff's and Steinach's operations are rarely if ever performed today. Thyroid extract, of course, cures myxoedema, but has little other action on the elderly. Iodides are probably useless and ultraviolet light actually produces premature skin ageing. Radioactivity is always dangerous and even mud baths are temporarily out of fashion.

Perhaps the greatest contribution Dr. Lorand made to the ideas prevalent in the history of rejuvenation was a warning against gluttony. This was echoed more flamboyantly and more profitably by Gaylord Hauser some years later. Hauser was in many ways an architypal rejuvenationist. Personally charming, healthy-looking and virile, he promised a similar constitution to those who followed his principles. His patients were famous people and included Greta Garbo, the Duchess of Windsor, Queen Alexandra of Yugoslavia, Norma Shearer and Douglas Fairbanks. Lady Elsie Mendl was a star in Hauser's rejuvenational firmament and could even stand on her head at the age of ninety-four.

Gaylord Hauser's method consists of diets made up from "wonder foods", often elaborated and marketed by Hauser himself, for example "Hollywood Slimming tea", "Healthwise", "Sipp" and "Nu-veg-Sal". They were usually of the low-calorie type, but sometimes he enthused over high potassium, sodium and calcium diets. He came very close toward Lorand's credo when he proposed in 1932 that everyone who wanted to live longer should retire to a quiet spot in the house with a tin-opener and a stock of his patent foods, for a frugal *Gesundheitstag*, which really just turned out to be a one day a week starvation episode. Rejuvenation "cures" of this ilk are, of course, common enough in the modern Health Farm arrangements.

11

Maintenance Rejuvenation

Although there is plenty of evidence that many of the aspects of rejuvenation dealt with in previous chapters are active enough, albeit in small measure, in the cities of the world today, perhaps the most exciting and most hopeful might be referred to as maintenance rejuvenation. This has been worked out against the background of normal, conventional public health practice. By maintenance rejuvenation an analogy is purposely made with the machine that has to be inspected and attended to in various ways at regular intervals if maximum efficiency is to be maintained.

Of course there are certain aspects of healthy living that have to be dealt with by the patient and the medical profession which stand outside the concept of rejuvenation, if this word is taken to mean a return of activity, health and happiness in later years. Far too many are stricken down in late middle life with diseases that are partially preventable today and may be wholly preventable tomorrow.

Delegates to the Sixth International Congress of Gerontology at Stockholm in 1963 heard a leading Danish expert suggest that the normal lifespan should be 100 to 120 years. An American expert is on record as suggesting a lifespan of 90 to 115 years might well be expected,[112] and even the opinion of a conservative medical biologist, one of the few scientists in this country much involved in the biology of ageing, believes that death from senescence rather than disease processes can be expected to occur between the age of 75 and 100.[18]

Exactly how far we are falling behind these seriously-expressed opinions becomes apparent when one considers that in 1961, the last year for which full figures are available, the average life span for men in England is 68 years (US 67). Women on the average live a longer life, that is, to the age of about 75.

The various reasons for the extraordinary health paradox that the average man of fifty has an expectation of life only two years longer in the 1960s than his father did in the 1930s, despite the fantastic advances in medical and surgical skills made possible largely by the antibiotic age and the pharmaceutical revolution has been dealt with elsewhere.[79] The contribution that coronary thrombosis, various forms of cancer, peptic ulcerations, accidents and chronic bronchitis make towards these dismal figures cannot be stressed further here.

The idea of maintenance rejuvenation, in contrast to many other ideas on the subject, has largely hailed from a very respectable part of the medical world, for few would argue that there is anything remotely flamboyant or exciting about public health and hygiene. This being the case it is hardly surprising that maintenance rejuvenation remains closely tied to the sociological and political principles of that world, and in certain ways has to suffer because of its origin. Because public health and hygiene evolved due to pressure of public opinion brought to bear on local authorities by men like Thomas Southwood Smith and Sir Edwin Chadwick in England, and through Lemuel Shattuck in the US, this speciality, within the framework of general medicine, has always had close municipal or local state ties. This being so it often takes on a rather parochial aspect that varies from place to place and country to country.

Originally in the middle of the nineteenth century the embryonic hygiene administrators and workers in the field were mainly concerned with the proper burial of the dead, the provision of clean, safe water, the construction of sewers and the removal of house refuse.

"They called for sick returns, for death rolls. They worked for the abolition of cesspools, of proper drains, of removable dust-bins. They clamoured above everything else, for new houses. They condemned filthy dairies, reeking slaughter-houses, and tainted oyster-beds. They penetrated into basement sweat shops and school lavatories. They exposed the adulteration of food and the sophistication of drugs. They protested at the free sale of poisons and opiates".[113] Gradually in this country the public health service welded itself into a more or less homogenous unit with its own hierarchy and discipline. The Public Health Acts of 1875 made it obligatory for every urban and rural area in Britain to appoint a Medical Officer of Health and similar legislation even-tually found favour throughout the civilized world.

During the early decades of the twentieth century doctors employed by local authorities busied themselves mainly with the health of the expectant mother, the newborn child and the school child. As such they were fulfilling an extremely valuable function, inasmuch as large numbers of the population could not, or did not take advantage of what was available from the general run of medical practice at this time. Gradually, however, in most European countries at any rate, state-subsidized medical insurance schemes or Health Services have taken over much of the raw material for which the local authority medical services previously existed. This being the case, those with progressive outlooks have directed their attention to another underprivileged age group, notably the elderly. And as such have unwittingly involved them-selves in the controversial subject of rejuvenation.

From the very beginning public health doctors have had to fight hard to do the work they felt was important. In the middle of the nineteenth century they often had to pit their wits against the vested interests of ratepayers, and the property-owning classes. Today they often have to wrestle with health committees that may hold extremely conservative ideas as to how to advise the ratepayers to spend their money. Public health doctors are usually single-minded and energetic. Occasionally their personalities carry them to the forefront in their chosen sphere of work, and they stand out as remarkable people preaching a remarkable gospel.

The gospel under consideration, that of maintenance rejuvenation, rests on two important procedures. First of all an extremely complete examination of the patient, and his medical history, in depth. Exactly what is meant by this phrase will be explained more fully later. Secondly it embraces the treatment, by reference to other branches of medicine if need be, of any disclosed physical illnesses and the correction of any deficiency diseases that are discovered.

To be effective the medical examination in depth, sometimes referred to as routine health check, or checkup, is in its essentials a team operation and far beyond the general capabilities and facilities available to the average practitioner. It is essential too that such an examination should be an "all at one time in one place" affair if it is to appeal to the tired and the elderly. As such it can be operated well from a local authority clinic in conjunction with an adjacent pathological laboratory.

An example of the type of medical examination in depth that not only indicates abnormalities discovered but provides a baseline from which amelioration or degeneration can be noted as time passes has been presented by Dr. John Maddison of the Experimental Clinic for older people at Teddington in London. At the time of writing he and his colleagues have done more than 450 first examinations and 7,500 subsequent follow-up consultations over a period of five years. Patients find their way to the clinic either through the activity of health visitors or local doctors. They do not come complaining of a specific symptom or disease, neither are they asked what they think they are suffering from, but are approached from the point of view of whether, as far as can be physically ascertained, they are as healthy as they could be for their age.

The physical examination in depth covers the following points. A general medical history is taken, and special trained personnel or doctors carry out a battery of screening tests. Weight, height (sitting and standing), pulse rate, temperature, skinfold thicknesses and thigh muscle strength and grip strength are measured. Any muscle distortions are noted, the reaction time is tested as are the blood pressure and urine. A sample of blood is sent to the laboratory, an electrocardiogram is taken and the respiratory exchange is measured. A photographic colour transparency under standard conditions is taken for comparison assessment at a later date.

Then various special sense investigations are conducted. The eyes are examined with reference to the condition of cornea, the intra-ocular tension, the lens is examined for cataract and the vitreous for opacities. Pupillary reactions are noted and then a full visual assessment with and without glasses is made. The visual fields are mapped out and the retina examined ophthalmologically, with reference to the condition of the vessels and other fundal structures.

The ears are then examined, wax is removed if necessary, the drum observed for abnormalities, the hearing being later assessed by audiometry and voice tests.

The physical examination continues along normal lines with specific accent on signs of bodily ageing. It is noted whether the general physique shows features of obesity, flabbiness or oedema, or whether thinness, wasting or shrinking of the stature, a bent back or head, slouching of the shoulders or bending of the knees are present. The gait is observed and any special characteristics noted.

The condition of the hair on the scalp, in the axilla, on the arms, body, genitals and legs is observed, and whether the eyebrows are bushy or thin, present or absent or scanty is recorded. The eyelids themselves are scrutinized for signs of "crows feet", puffiness, droopiness. Any characteristic "hooding" and the presence or absence of tear overflow from the eyes is recorded and the characteristic of the conjunctiva is also noted and described. The nose is examined with reference to the condition of the septum and the nasal turbinates and the meatus are inspected for any discharge, congestion or obstruction. The teeth and dentures come in for scrutiny next and the condition of the tongue, throat and voice assessed.

As far as head, limbs and trunk mobility and structure are concerned, very specialized and detailed tests are carried out far beyond what might be considered necessary in, for example, an examination for life insurance. Although the general condition of the musculature of the neck, arms and legs is important, the skin of the scalp, forehead, face, neck, shoulders, arm, chest, abdomen, perineum, thigh, leg and foot are also examined carefully and any dryness, coarseness, wrinkled character, inelastic quality and hairlessness, pigmentation or petechial quality is recorded.

The bones and joints of the neck, shoulder, elbow, wrist, fingers, spine, hip, knee, ankle and toes are also carefully examined and aches and pains, rheumatic nodes, swelling, thickening, deformity, limitation of movement as well as the classical signs of rheumatoid or osteoarthritis are noted if present. The legs are examined for varicose veins and feet for bunions, hammer toe, corns, callosities, flat foot and nail deformities. The limb reflexes are also assessed.

The heart and lungs come in for very thorough testing of a classical type and the abdomen is examined for tumours and ruptures. A rectal examination, with special reference to the prostate glands is carried out in the case of men, and in woman a vaginal examination and a careful inspection of the breasts completes the testing. As might be expected, the whole procedure takes several hours and suitable pauses for resting, light snacks and hot drinks breaks up the rather athletic medical routine.

This particular examination in depth, so necessary before anything in the nature of replacement rejuvenation proper takes place, is carried out, at the Teddington Clinic, in a converted building that is far from ideal, and the system is a triumph of British "make do with what you can get" medicine. Dr. Maddison has given his ideas on a more ideal condition of work. Although these are far advanced from the present arrangements, they can hardly be considered elaborate or exotic when judged by European or US clinical standards and will be detailed later.

Nevertheless the results obtained at Teddington produce a wealth of information. First of all they provide a valuable health and biological age baseline for each individual patient. Any treatment subsequently given can naturally be related to this baseline. Secondly the results give an idea of the number of physical disabilities carried by each patient that are, by and large, in their summation producing the clinical picture of biological age, seen in that patient. In other words *apparent age* and *wealth of disability* become substantially related to one another.

It is doubtful if anyone who had not studied the problem previously would be able to make even an approximate guess at the multiplicity of disability that comes to light from an examination in depth or a random sample of older people. Of the first 360 patients that attended Maddison's clinic (128 men, 232 women)—fifty-eight of whom were under 60 years old—nobody was found to have nothing wrong with them. Only eight had one disability, 139 patients suffered from two to ten, diagnosible diseases, 119 from eleven to fourteen such illnesses, while sixty-one patients were found to have between fifteen and seventeen things wrong. Five people had over twenty separate disabilities to carry.

Critics may argue that many of these disabilities are trivial. Admittedly 288 patients out of the 360 were found to have incorrect glasses or eye defects, and 250 had troubles with hearing, mostly due to wax being present in the ears. These disabilities, however, are particularly remedial and can make a tremendous contribution to a patient's wellbeing if treated. Many of the disabilities discovered too are beyond cure in the present state of knowledge. 105 cases of coronary heart disease, 262 of arterial diseases came to light, but even in these cases amelioration can often be effected with subsequent improvement in outlook for patients by adequate treatment.

Many of the disabilities discovered by a physical examination in depth are, however, very much within the range of twentieth-century therapeutics, and a number of these can be so efficiently treated that the word cure is not inappropriate. It is in these cases that there can be a definite and reasonable reduction in biological age effected—a rejuvenation brought about by modern medicine.

There are several broad fields of therapy in which this can occur, the first of which comes under the heading of Nutrition. Maddison found that over a third of his patients suffered from a nutritional deficiency of one kind or another. It is fashionable to look upon deficiency diseases as being due to one specific deficiency in the diet, for example scurvy brought about by deficiency of vitamin C, or pellegra, being due to niacin deficiency. However, it is doubtful if deficiency of a single nutrient substance ever clinically brings about a deficiency disease in practice. The absence of one essential nutrient sometimes brings about initially some upset in the complex business of food digestion, or assimilation. This in turn produces inadequate absorption or utilization of other foodstuff, and what may have started biologically at one point becomes clinically a multiple deficiency syndrome.

In many cases the diagnosis of malnutrition, defined by Maddison as impairment of the functional efficiency of the body systems that can be corrected by better feeding, has to be sought out as scientifically and assiduously as that of any other disease. It is important to remember too that the history of a defective diet is not always well given by those whose intellectual and social qualities have been impaired by that diet, and when it is given it can often be unreliable. Then laboratory and clinical tests must be carried out. Biochemical tests for subnormal levels of proteins, vitamins and minerals can give valuable information as can the detection of abnormal metabolites.

The conception of malnutrition of the elderly is fundamentally one of protein deficiency, brought about by eating habits that include a regime of no breakfast, a very small lunch of meat and vegetables, a bread and jam tea and a liquid supper. Sometimes if the diet is characterized by carbohydrate fillers the malnutrition of obesity supervenes to complicate the picture.

Generally speaking, Maddison finds the following clinical features present in patients suffering from this malnutrition of the ageing. There are subjective feelings of fatigue, sleepiness by day and insomnia at night. Often there is a diagnostic irritableness or querulousness. Appetite is generally poor and sustained effort either physical or mental is difficult. There are vague disturbances of sensation, and of mood, that progress in some cases to neurosis or even psychosis. On examination there is either the paunchy obesity of excessive carbohydrate intake or the thin, wasted, frail and flabby, slow moving and clumsy wasting of the elderly.

Skin changes are highly characteristic. Usually this is excessively dry and scaly with a tendency to desquamation, and is due to deficiency in sebum and sweat secretion. Patches of pigmentation of haemorrhageic spots are common, with a tendency to easy bruising. Elasticity of all tissues is diminished profoundly and there is a tendency to angular stomatitis around the mouth, eczema-intertrigo at skin creases and the chronic thickening of the skin at areas of friction known as lichenification. The hair in protein deficiency is typically grey, thin and lustreless, while the nails are dry, slow-growing and ridged, often showing opaque white bands. The musculature is poor and inefficient while the bones are thin and brittle. Apart from these general signs Maddison describes various specific features in the general medical examination as well as changes in urine analysis and blood chemistry, X-rays and electrocardiograph tracings.

Protein malnutrition is not a static condition. Unless it is tackled energetically it becomes associated with, and aggravates, various other physical disabilities, for example generalized tissue loss, osteoporosis, anaemia and more specific vitamin deficiencies. The first step therefore in rejuvenating the elderly is to improve dietary protein intake. Elderly folk finding themselves in a state of protein malnutrition mainly do so for three reasons: poverty, ignorance of what is good for them to eat, and apathy. Often these three factors conspire together to reduce the stamina and fitness of patients. A poor income is liable to be associated with old-fashioned or worn-out kitchen equipment that is difficult to clean and use for cooking. Meals, therefore, tend to become excessively simple and unappetizing. If the shops are some distance away, dentures are ill-fitting, or there is no one to cook for anyway, apathy tends to rule the roost.

Maddison believes that older people need a higher proportion of protein in their diet than those in middle age, and this works out at about four ounces of lean meat daily or its equivalent in eggs, milk, fish or cheese. This is about three times as much as has previously been considered necessary for older people, and represents a considerable sum of money when measured in terms of pensionable salary in many cases. In 1963, shopping in the most economical circumstances, the protein requirements of the elderly alone were estimated to cost about 21s. 6d. per week in these islands. Since then most prices have outstripped pensions.

Once the patients have been placed in a state of protein stability the replacement regime then turns its attention towards correcting any mineral and vitamin deficiencies. These are mainly responsible for the diseases of osteoporosis and anaemia in the elderly. If it were necessary to point out one illness that contributes more to the impression of senility than any other, osteoporosis would be the natural choice. It is a major disease of the elderly and is largely responsible for the bent and shrunken appearance of many of our senior citizens. Quite often its symptoms and signs follow an illness or operation and in its earliest stages it causes the "old man's buffalo hump" in the neck. The bodies of the lower cervical and upper thoracic vertebrae become wedge-shaped and so the head comes forward while the neck "humps" backwards. Sometimes these changes become more pronounced and the whole spine becomes kinked and deformed. Naturally enough these vertebral changes often produce unpleasant symptoms. Commonly there is aching of the back, pains in the limbs, especially in the shins. Arthritic changes often take place in the joints around the deformed bones. Spontaneous fractures of bone occur in severe cases.

Osteoporosis, sometimes referred to as osteopenia, is a disease entity that is diagnosed largely on clinical grounds, as X-ray changes in bones in the disease cannot be usually demonstrated until there is a 30 to 50 per cent reduction in bone mass. Bone biopy can provide an earlier diagnosis but is a traumatic procedure not kindly accepted by elderly people. Experts disagree as to the exact aetiology of osteoporosis but the consensus of opinion is that it is due to an imbalance of the internal steroid environment of the patient. Maddison believes that it is part of a multiple deficiency syndrome of older people and can be effectively treated with a combination of calcium, magnesium, fluorine, vitamin D, citrate and an anabolic steroid, provided a full protein diet is given. Sometimes he finds that thyroxine is also necessary for effective treatment. Most important, improvement after a few months' treatment is "quite striking".

Not all physicians are as enthusiastic about the effects of treatment of osteoporosis however. At an International Symposium on protein metabolism held at Leyden in 1962 the consensus of opinion seemed to be that subjective improvement could be effected in fairly advanced cases by means of anabolic steroid therapy, but that no change in calcium accretation rate could be demonstrated in bones, and that these findings cast doubt on the value of anabolic steroids in the treatment of osteopenia.[114] It must be stressed, however, that Maddison underlines *early* protein stabilization and energetic treatment with minerals and vitamins as described above, together with hormone treatment can largely prevent severe osteoporic states becoming established.

Part of the regime for prevention of osteoporosis is the correction of any anaemic tendency in the patient. Anaemia in its own right is very prevalent in old people and approximately a third of all the patients treated at the Teddington Clinic were anaemic when they first arrived. In all probability anaemia is an intrinsic part of the malnutrition syndrome of the elderly. In some cases malabsorption of iron is responsible for the condition. Chronic blood loss due to intestinal bleeding can have the same effect. The large majority of anaemia diagnosed is of a simple iron-deficiency type, but other, macrocytic, anaemias are encountered. Maddison believes that vitamin B12 and folic-acid deficiencies are present in his patients long before the classical signs of macrocytic (pernicious) anaemia become obvious, and he has observed that *senile lentigo*, pigmented spots about 1 to 5 millimetres in diameter that occur on the hands, forearms, temples and forehead of the elderly, disappear after three to four months' treatment with folic acid.

Other vitamin deficiencies are also corrected wherever signs of them are seen as part of healthy maintenance therapy. Vitamins are given in larger doses than is usual during early life, due to the possibility of poor absorption taking place in the elderly.

A systematic attempt to diagnose and treat any hormone deficiencies in the elderly completes what might be described as the physical side of maintenance rejuvenation, and perhaps the most common hormone deficiency disease in the elderly is that of thyroid hormone. Even in its florid form in the clinical picture of a patient suffering from thyroid deficiency or myxoedema there are certain features reminiscent of bodily changes that we refer to commonly as senile. The myxoedema patient is intellectually slow, dull and apathetic. There is a disinclination to attempt any mental or physical effort. A curious easy-going emotionless attitude affects these patients who do not seem to care about how they look or how they spend their waking hours that are always punctuated with periods of day sleep. Myxoedemics feel the cold rather badly and tend to wrap up excessively and their dry, sallow, puffy skin feels cold to the touch. The slowness of these patients' nervous systems is reflected in the characteristic bodily movement which is at the same time ponderous, timid and clumsy. Together with these locomotion characteristics goes a facial expression that denotes a miserable stupidity. The face tends to be puffy, the hair thin and lustreless and frequently in both sexes there is temporal baldness and loss of the eyebrows, especially in the outer third. Body hair elsewhere is sparse or absent.

Myxoedematous patients are often deaf, speak infrequently with a low, croaking voice and have a poor appetite incongruous with their generalized obesity. They are sexually apathetic, and usually impotent. Physical examination of the myxoedematous patient reveals characteristic changes and the diagnosis can be confirmed by a number of biochemical and haemotological tests. The electrocardiogram also shows specific changes.

Many old people become myxoedematous so insidiously that neither they nor their relatives or companions notice the changes, which are once again written off as being due to old age. Maddison believes that many older people do, in fact, suffer from thyroid deficiency long before the classical picture of myxoedema develops, and there would seem little reason to doubt him on this score, for over a third of his original series of patients had thyroid deficiency. Many of the symptoms and signs of established myxoedema can be reversed by treatment with thyroid hormone and the complications in the untreated case that include heart failure and virtual imbecility completely avoided.

The final main deficiency disease that masquerades as ill health,

Maddison feels, is due to lack of another group of internal secretions, known as the anabolic steroids. To a certain extent this aspect of the rejuvenation is an extension of earlier work carried out by the Steinach school. (*see* chapter 9.) The steroids are a complex group of organic chemicals, more or less closely related to one another, that are found in animal and plant tissues. As far as our subject is concerned the anabolic steroids are chemical substances either occurring naturally in the body or those which can be manufactured in the biochemists' laboratory that have a body-building or anabolic effect. Examples of naturally occurring anabolic steroids are testosterone in the male and oestrogen in the female. In both sexes substances produced in the cortex of the adrenal glands also have profound anabolic effects.

As previously stressed in chapter 9 the sex hormone steroids have an important effect on the appearance, biological age and behaviour of both man and the experimental animal. They also, together with the adrenal steroids, promote protein anabolism, increase the growth of muscle and effect the muscle to fat relationships and proportions throughout the body. Effective levels of the anabolic steroids throughout the body improve muscular strength and also have profound psychological effects. They are also generally thought to maintain libido, and promote a sense of wellbeing. As previously mentioned there is a relationship between their presence in normal amounts in the blood stream and calcium maintenance in the bones.

In normal people the available anabolic steroids gradually diminish as the years go by. Taking the androgens as an example, most men have measurably diminished blood androgen by the time they are fifty. Between the age of sixty and seventy they have lost approximately two-thirds and between seventy and eighty, three-quarters of what they possessed at the age of twenty-five.

Maddison maintains that anabolic steroid deficiency is characterized by a tendency to easy fatigue, failing muscular strength, loss of muscle substance and general tissue wasting that adds up to loss of weight in later years. There is also a characteristic ageing appearance of the facial skin, hooded eyebrows, crows feet and deeply lined cheeks, together with a scraggy neck that epitomizes early senility. Sexual apathy, loss of body hair, certain characteristic emotional and psychological problems are also frequently present.

To see to what extent these apparent signs of old age were in fact specific signs of anabolic steroid deficiency, a clinical trial was conducted. This was not the much-trusted and valuable double blind trial in which no one, doctor, patient, nurse or assessor knows who is receiving the drug under trial, but merely a clinical test as to response to treatment. One hundred and forty-four patients suffering from clinically obvious steroid deficiency were carefully matched together in pairs, with reference to age and sex. Their ages ranged from forty-nine to eighty-seven. As might be expected, as well as the steroid deficiency presumed, many had other physical disabilities including artery disease, hypertension, coronary thrombosis, arthritis, asthma, bronchitis, peptic ulcer as well as other deficiency syndromes such as generalized malnutrition, obesity or anaemia. Some had thyroid deficiency and senile skin diseases.

In both groups, as was normal practice, glandular or malnutrition syndromes were corrected but in only one group synthetic anabolic steroids were given in addition. Maddison found the clinical difference between the two groups "unmistakable". They looked younger than their matched controls. The facial lines practically disappeared. Exercise tasks that previously had been too much for them they now took in their stride. Grip tests and leg strength tests improved strikingly. Mental attitudes were changed for the better and in some cases lost virility was restored. Usually if emaciation was produced, an increase of 7 pounds took place over the four years involved in the trial, although those who had signs of obesity either lost weight or remained at constant weight, fat being replaced by muscle. Measured elasticity of the skin improved and serial photographs confirmed a more youthful aspect and appearance.

One of the unique aspects of the striking and sustained rejuvenation produced by the maintenance regime advocated by Maddison is the difficulty involved in persuading patients to swallow a multiplicity of tablets daily. This was overcome by the simple expedient of combining them all into a powder. Of course each powder being tailor-made to fit each individual's assessed deficiency, tends to be formulated differently, although obviously a certain grouping together of similar patients permits some "stock mixtures" being made up. Patients are asked to take their dose of powder in the morning in the form of a milky drink, or with maize oil. In this way the large majority of people can be relied upon to take their medicine and do not alter treatment routines due to sudden and often inexplicable dislikes of certain pills or tablets met with so frequently in clinical medicine.

Dr. John Maddison is clearly quite convinced that his methods for "keeping the Old Folks Young" work. Obviously those who live in the catchment area of his clinic believe so too. From being a small, relatively unknown organization with few patients, it has grown in a few years quite prodigiously and the number of the staff employed, both medical and paramedical, has had to be substantially augmented. There is a waiting list for new patients, and frequent requests from patients living outside the local authority area involved who have to be refused routinely. Little support has come from the body of the medical profession but any doctor who takes the trouble to visit the clinic cannot fail to be impressed.

A consultant geriatrician summed up his verdict on maintenance rejuvenation in the following words:

What you [Maddison] are doing is to pick out, treat, minimize and alleviate those defects and deteriorations which are amenable to treatment, such as the anaemias, hypothyroidism, anabolic steroid deficiency, foot defects and visual defects. You recognize other defects and observe and note them, but in our present state of knowledge you cannot cure or reverse them. But you try various experiments and tests and therapeutic measures and continue your research in the hope of finding better methods. And all this is to the good. I see that this clinic steps right out in front of the general practitioner service which waits for the sick patient to attend with his textbook diagnosable disease: and still further in front of the hospital service with its load of irremediable cases and wrecks which we can do nothing for at the far end of the scale.[115]

Although certain other local health authorities have followed in Teddington's footsteps to some extent, there is no great enthusiasm for further extensions of this apparently extremely efficient method of twentieth-century rejuvenation. Based as it is around an examination of the apparently "not ill" patient, it comes under the general umbrella heading of the routine medical checkup, a procedure viewed with a variable amount of suspicion by doctors everywhere and with more than average suspicion by the profession in Great Britain.

Despite mounting evidence that proves apparently without a shadow of doubt that many diseases, including several aspects of malignancy, can have their mortality substantially stemmed by earlier diagnosis, they believe that much psychological and phobic illness is fostered by the procedure. Recently in the US there are signs that this issue may well be settled scientifically. A health screening programme on the West Coast has been set up that screens some 4,000 people a month at some twenty centres, a procedure which, suitably computerized, takes about two hours and costs around thirty dollars. It is also taking part in a controlled study involving some 10,000 patients. Morbidity, mortality and total expenditure in terms of money spent on health are being compared between groups investing in routine screening procedures and those who make use of medical aid "on demand" when it is personally required.

As previously mentioned, the clinic that operates maintenance rejuvenation at Teddington is limited with regard to both equipment and space. Over the years Maddison has had time to ponder over the sort of clinic that should ideally be available to all older people in an area the size of an average London borough. He feels that the clinic should be planned around five suites of clinical consulting rooms, each with its individual examination room. Nearby and probably communicating with these suites there should be a special darkened room where examination of the eye, nose, throat and ear can be carried out with the aid of all necessary special equipment. There should be a laboratory in which physical tests of a physiological nature can be carried out, and a biochemical department with facilities for blood-testing and urine analysis situated with an adjoining urine collection room. A suitably staffed dental suite, two chiropody surgeries, a physiotherapy room and a therapeutic swimming-bath, together with a small X-ray room and X-ray developing dark room completes the medical requirements.

Such a clinic ideally has functions outside the purely diagnostic. Health education for the elderly is considered as important as that for the expectant mother, and so a meeting room, together with projection facilities, should be available. Due to the principle of "one time, one place", thought so essential in this work, an adequate waiting room, refreshment bar, food sales bar and shop, together with a staff room and canteen are essential. The provision of therapeutic substances necessitates a small dispensary and, clearly, adequate office accommodation and record storage must be met.

Routine and convention dictate that space must also be put aside within the scheme of things for toilets, cleaners' room, workshop, boiler room and a car park for at least twenty cars. All in all this would represent a capital investment of some magnitude and perhaps this is the real reason for the most promising rejuvenation method of the twentieth century being pigeonholed almost indefinitely—in the hope, perhaps, that something cheaper will eventually be unearthed that will give us the answer to longer and more active lives in the years to come.

Always there have been those who look upon a step forward with great suspicion, and see potential disaster in every advance of science. As far as rejuvenation is concerned we seem to be quite near a scientific breakthrough that will change all our lives and alter society profoundly. A leading gerontologist feels that all that is necessary for this to come to pass is money. This, he says, should be used to recruit a research team headed by three biologists of Nobel Prize quality, who, if determined to probe the problems of ageing with assiduity, will ensure that quite soon the average man and woman's expectation of vigorous human life could be extended five or ten years past the Biblical three score years and ten.[116]

The broad principles involved in this postulated breakthrough would be to extend the field of Geriatrics and improve on treatment of the disabilities of old age and palliate the loss of health associated with it and this approximates closely to maintenance therapy. More exciting perhaps is the possibility of a concentrated attack on the biomechanics of the "clock" that times the decline of vigour in the individual. Once these mechanics are understood suitable and useful regulation adjustments will be feasible. Biology, the essential science of life, seems to be poised for a tremendous advance in basic knowledge that will match similar twentieth-century advances in nuclear physics. "The third great alchemical dream, the 'Elixir of Life' seems almost ready to be bottled".[117] One can only hope that when this happens the flavour will be thoroughly acceptable.

Bibliographical Notes

[CHAPTER ONE]

1. Codellas, P. S. *Rejuvenations and Satyricons of Yesterday.* Annals of Medical History, vol. VI, 1934

[CHAPTER TWO]

2. Garrison, Fielding H. *An Introduction to the History of Medicine.* Saunders: 1929
3. Roberts, Morley. *Folklore,* vol. XXVII. 1916
4. Blum, Richard and Eva. *Health and Healing in Rural Greece.* Stanford University Press: 1965
5. Gutherie, Douglas. *A History of Medicine.* Nelson: 1945
6. Ellis, Havelock. *Studies in the Psychology of Sex.* Random House: 1936
7. Haggard, Howard W. *Devils, Drugs and Doctors.* Heinemann: 1929
8. Grieve, M. *A Modern Herbal.* Jonathan Cape: 1931
9. Davenport, John. *Aphrodisiacs and Anti-aphrodisiacs.* London, privately printed: 1869
10. Grigson, Geoffrey. *The Englishman's Flora.* Phoenix House: 1958
11. Leyel, C. F. *Nutritious Herbs.* Faber: 1948
12. Frazer, J. G. *The Magic Art,* vol. II. Macmillan: 1911
13. Loudon, J. C. *Encyclopaedia of Plants.* Longmans: 1841
14. Burton, Sir Richard. *Perfumed Garden of Shaykh Nefzawi* (trans.). Panther Books: 1963
15. Bay, Pilaff and Douglas, Norman. *Venus in the Kitchen.* Heinemann: 1952
16. Clair, Colin. *Of Herbs and Spices.* Abelard-Schuman: 1961
17. Grigson, Geoffrey. *A Herbal of Sorts.* Phoenix House: 1959
18. Comfort, Alex. *Biology of Senescence.* Routledge and Kegan Paul: 1956
19. Sushruta. *English Translations of Sushruta Samita.* Wilkins Press, Calcutta: 1911
20. Veith, Ilza. *Modern Medicine.* November, 1961

[CHAPTER THREE]

21. Culpepper, Nicholas. *London Dispensatory.* 1679

22. Quincey, John. *The Compleat English Dispensatory.* 1722
23. Licht, Hans. *Sexual Life in Ancient Greece.* Routledge: 1932
24. Virgil. *Aeneid: Book IV*
25. Frazer, J. G. *Pausanias's Description of Greece.* Macmillan: 1898
26. Walsh, James. *The Thirteenth, Greatest of Centuries.* Fordham University Press: 1937
27. Chin P'Ing Mei. *The Golden Lotus.* Clement Egerton, Routledge: 1939
28. Walton, Alan Hall. *Aphrodisiacs.* Associated Booksellers, Connecticut: 1958
29. Sollman, Torald. *A Manual of Pharmacology.* W. B. Saunders Company: 1957
30. Lély, Gilbert. *The Marquis de Sade* (trans. Alec Brown). Elek: 1961

[CHAPTER FOUR]
31. Wright, Lawrence. *Clean and Decent.* Routledge and Kegan Paul: 1960
32. Masson, P. *Larouse Encyclopaedia of Mythology.* Batchworth Press: 1959
33. *MD* magazine, Vol. 5. September, 1961
34. Zarncke, F. *Der Priester Johannés.* Leipzig: 1876
35. Yule, Sir Henry. *Encyclopaedia Britannica* 9th edition
36. Brinton, D. G. *Notes on the Floridian Peninsula.* Joseph Sabin, Philadelphia: 1859
37. Reniers, Perceval. *The Springs of Virginia, 1775–1900.* University of North Carolina Press: 1941
38. Clement of Alexandria. *Paedagogus* Book III, Chapter V.
39. Addison, William. *English Spas.* B. T. Batsford Ltd., 1951
40. Rowzee, Lodwick. *The Queene's Wells.* 1632.
41. Veteran, A. *Hints to the Sick, the Lame and the Lazy, or Passages in the Life of a Hydropathist.* John Oliver: 1857
42. Lane, Richard J. *Life at the Water Cure.* Longmans: 1846
43. Jameson, Eric. *Natural History of Quackery.* Michael Joseph: 1961
44. Bell, John. *A Treatise of Baths.* Barrington & Haswell, Philadelphia: 1850
45. Johnson, Edward. *The Domestic Practice of Hydropathy.* Simpkin, March & Co.: 1856
46. Weber, Hermann and Weber, F. Pakes. *The Spas and Mineral Waters of Europe:* 1896

[CHAPTER FIVE]
47. Trimmer, Eric J. *Some Quack Contributions to Orthodox Medicine.* Roche Image: 1965

48. *Annals.* Royal College of Physicians, London.

49. *Receit showing the way to make his most Excellent Medicine called Aurum Potabile.* Printed by William Cooper: 1683

50. Thompson, C. J. S. *The Quacks of Old London.* Bretanos, London: 1928

51. Angelo, Henry. *Reminiscences.* Colburn and Bentley: 1830

52. Graham, James. *The Guardian of Health, Long Life and Happiness.* Undated pamphlet

53. Graham, James. *The Whole Art of Preventing and Curing Disease.* Undated pamphlet. London. 'Printed for the people and by the Rosy Heralds of Health distributed. 2d.'

54. Lysons, Daniel. *Collectionanae.* 1660–1840.

55. Graham, James. *Il Corvito Amorosa* a lecture delivered at the Temple of Hymen, 1782

56. *More Secret Remedies.* British Medical Association: 1912

57. *Nostrums and Quackery*, Vol. 2, American Medical Association: 1921

58. *Journal American Medical Association.* 25th October, 1919

59. *Nostrums and Quackery*, Vol. 1, American Medical Association: 1912

60. Brodum, William. *A Guide to Old Age and a Cure for the Indiscretions of Youth*

61. *Chicago Tribune.* 2nd November, 1913

62. *Nostrums and Quackery*, Vol. 2, Handbill of Wisconsin Medical Institute

63. *Nostrums and Quackery*, Vol. 3, American Medical Association

64. Gardner, Martin. *Fads and Fallacies in the Name of Science.* Dover Publications Incorporated, New York: 1957

[CHAPTER SIX]

65. Metchnikoff, Olga. *Life of Elie Metchnikoff.* Constable & Co., London: 1921

66. *Untersuchungen über die intracelluläre Verdanung Arbeiten zool.* Instituts zu Wien. V.Z.

67. Virchow's *Archiv.* Vol. 96

68. Metchnikoff, Elie. *Prolongation of Life.* Heinemann: 1907

69. *Gazette des Hopitaux.* 1904

70. *Accidents due a la Constipation prendant la Grossesse, l'Accouchement et les Suites de Couches.* Paris: 1902

[CHAPTER SEVEN]

71. Niehans, Paul. *Die Endokreinen Drüsen des Gehirns, Epiphyse und Hypophyse.* Hans Halen, Berne, Switzerland.

72. Niehans, Paul. *Introduction to Cellular Therapy*. Pageant Book Inc., New York: 1960.
73. Lambert, Gilbert. *Conquest of Age*. Souvenir Press, London: 1960
74. Niehans, Paul. *Cellular Therapy*. Ott Verlag Thun, Switzerland: 1964

[CHAPTER EIGHT]

75. Parhon, Professor C. I. *Die Therapeiwoche*, Vol. 8, No. 1.
76. Volles, Stanley F. *Today's Health*. March 1966
77. Aslan, Professor Anna. *Die Therapeiwoche*, Vol. 7, No. 12. 12th October, 1956
78. *British Medical Journal*. 28th November, 1959
79. Trimmer, Eric J. *Live Long, Stay Young*. George Allen & Unwin: 1965
80. *Research on Novocain therapy in Old Age*. Consultant's Bureau Inc.: 1959
81. *Bulletin Experimental Biology and Medicine*. U.S.S.R. No. 8: 1958
82. Kohlen, U. and Mampel, F. *Die Therapeiwoche*, Vol. 8, No. 1, October 1957
83. Gericke, Otto L. Lobb, Lois G. and Pardoll, Davis H. *Evolution of Procaine in Geriatric Patients in a Mental Hospital*. Journal of Clinical and Experimental Psychopathology. Vol. XXII, No. 1: March 1961

[CHAPTER NINE]

84. Brown-Séquard, Charles E. *Society de Biologique*. Paris: 1851 Vol. II
85. *Proceedings Royal Society* No. 297 Lancet: January 1875
86. Schmidt, Peter. *The Conquest of Old Age*. George Routledge: 1931
87. Steinach, Eugen & Loebel, Josef. *Sex and Life*. Faber & Faber: 1940
88. *Wenen Medizinische Wichenschrift*
89. Haire, Norman. *Rejuvenation*. Allen & Unwin: 1924.
90. Steinach, E. *Pflügers Archiv*. 144: 71. 1912
91. Steinach, E. *Intrbl. f. Physiol*. 27: 717: 1913
92. Steinach, E. *Archig. F. Entwicklungsmech*. 46: 553: 1920
93. Benjamin, Harry, M.D. *Steinach Therapy against Old Age*. American Medicine, December 1932
94. Benjamin, H. *Fifth International Congress of the World League for Sexual Reform*: 1932
95. Wheeler, Clayton E. *Medical Journal and Record*. 18th July, 1928
96. Walker, Kenneth M. *Commentary on Age*. Jonathan Cape: 1952
97. *Medical Journal and Record*. 187.28
98. *Medical Review of Reviews*. February 1928. Vol. XXXIV. No. 2.
99. *Journal American Medical Association*: 5th May, 1928

100. *New York Times.* 23.1.28
101. Walker, Kenneth M. *Practitioner.* Vol. 115, 1925
102. *Medical Review of Reviews.* Vol. 34. 1928, New York
103. *The Antiseptic.* A monthly Journal of Medicine and Surgery, May 1947 Vol. XLIV. No. 5
104. *Medical Review of Reviews.* (ibid.)

[CHAPTER TEN]
105. Koestler, Arthur. *The Sleepwalkers.* London: 1959
106. Inglis, Brian. *Fringe Medicine.* Faber & Faber: 1964
107. Jarvis, D. C. *Folk Medicine.* W. H. Allen: 1960
108. Maury, Marguerite. *The Secret of Life and Youth.* Macdonald, London: 1964
109. Bogomolets, Alexander A. *The Prolongation of Life.* (Trans. Peter V. Karpovich and Sonia Bleeker, Duell, Sloan and Pearce Inc., New York: 1946)
110. *MD* magazine. Borrowed Youth. September, 1961
111. Lorand, Arnold. *Life-Shortening Habits and Rejuvenation.* F. A. Davis, Philadelphia: 1923

[CHAPTER ELEVEN]
112. Stieglitz, Edward J. *The Second Forty Years.* Staples Press: 1949.
113. Turner, E. S. *Call the Doctor.* Michael Joseph: 1958
114. Dymling, J. F., Isaksson, B. and Sjogren, B. *Protein Metabolism Symposium.* Springer Verlog: 1962
115. Maddison, John. *How to Keep the Old Folks Young.* Privately Published. County Council of Middlesex
116. Comfort, Alex. *Trueman Wood Lecture.* Science and Longevity. R.S.A.: 1966
117. *Medical News.* 8th April, 1966

Index